INSTANT
Skincare

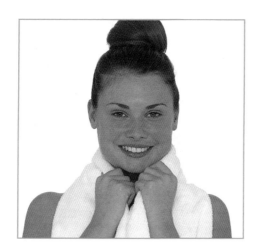

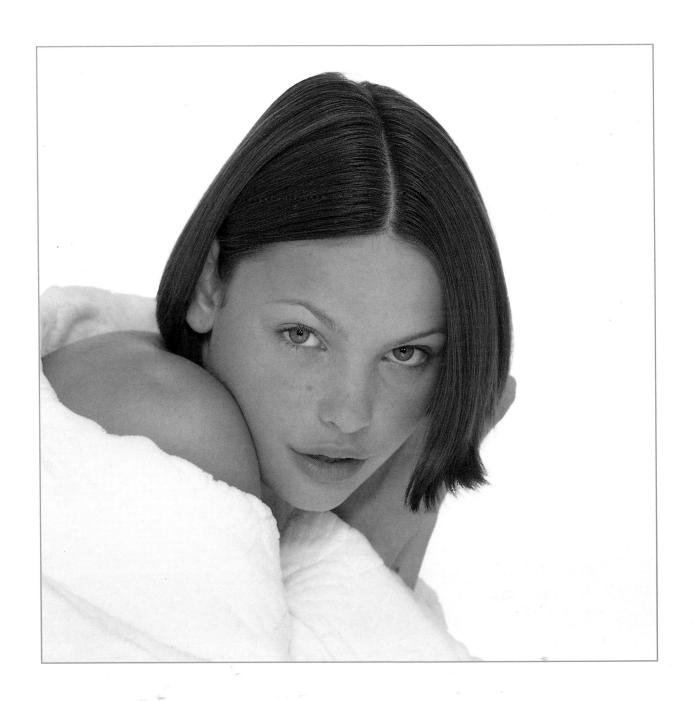

INSTANT
Skincare
How to have healthy, hassle-free skin

Sally Norton

Photography: Nick Cole

LORENZ BOOKS

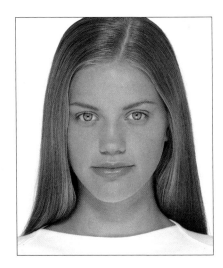

This edition first published in 1998 by Lorenz Books

Lorenz Books is an imprint of
Anness Publishing Limited
Hermes House
88–89 Blackfriars Road
London SE1 8HA

© 1998 Anness Publishing Limited

ISBN 1 85967 691 x

A CIP catalogue record for this book is available from the British Library

Publisher: Joanna Lorenz
Senior editor: Cathy Marriott
Designer: Ian Sandom
Additional text: Kate Shapland
Additional photography on pages 5, 7, 16, 17, 30, 44, 45, 46, 47, 48,
50 and 61 by Simon Bottomley
Photographs on pages 56-57 courtesy of Nivea

Printed in Singapore by Star Standard Industries Pte. Ltd.

1 3 5 7 9 10 8 6 4 2

Contents

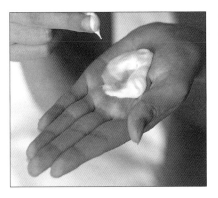 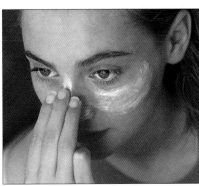 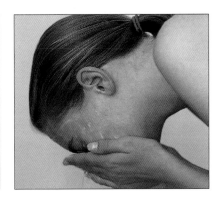

Beautiful Skin

Clear, soft and supple skin is one of the greatest beauty assets. While your actual skin type is determined by your genes, there's plenty you can do on a day-to-day basis to ensure it always looks as good as possible. Understanding how your skin functions will awaken you to its special needs. In this book we'll show you how to care for your own specific skin type. You can't neglect your complexion for months or years, then make up for it with expensive and intensive attention in the short term. You'll reap the benefits by regularly spending time and care on your skin. It's never too early or too late to follow a good skincare regime – because the results will last a lifetime.

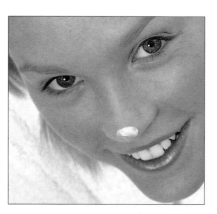

Above: Moisturizing your skin every day keeps it healthy and glowing.

Right: Remember to look after the skin on your whole body for all over beauty.

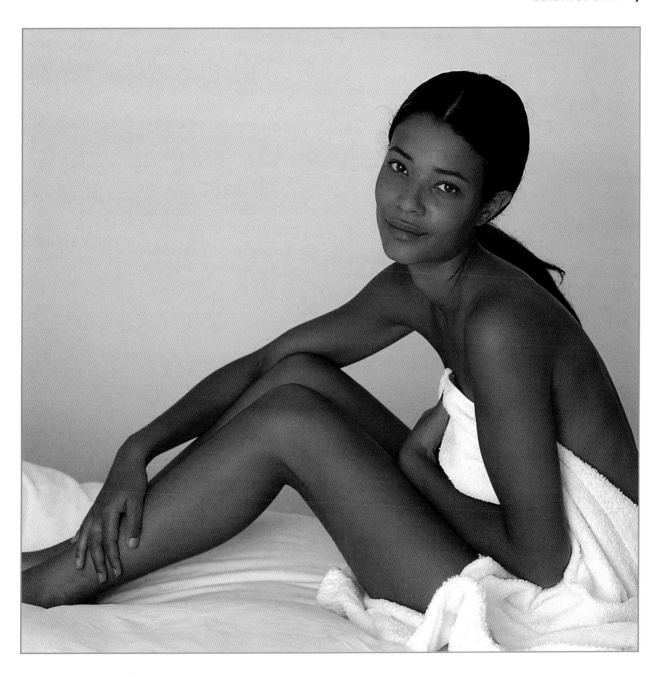

What is Skin?

Skin is your body's largest organ. Every woman can have beautiful skin no matter what her age, race or colouring. The secret is to understand how your skin functions and to treat it correctly. Your skin is made up of two main layers, called the epidermis and the dermis.

The epidermis

This is the top layer of skin and the one you can actually see. It protects your body from invasion and infection and helps to seal in moisture. It's built up of several layers of living cells that are then topped by sheets of dead cells. It's constantly growing, with new cells being produced at its base. They quickly die and are pushed up to the surface by the arrival of new ones. These dead cells eventually flake away, which means that every new layer of skin provides another chance to have a glowing complexion.

The lower levels of living cells are fed by the blood supply from underneath, whereas the upper dead cells only need water to ensure they are kept really plump and smooth.

The epidermis is responsible for your colouring, as it holds the skin's pigment. Its thickness varies from area to area – e.g. it's much thicker on the soles of your feet than on your eyelids.

The dermis

The dermis is the layer that lies underneath the epidermis, and it is composed entirely of living cells. It consists of bundles of tough fibres that give your skin its elasticity, firmness and strength. There are also blood vessels, which feed vital nutrients to these areas.

Whereas the epidermis can usually repair itself and make itself as good as new, the dermis will be permanently damaged by injury. The dermis also contains the following specialized organs:

Sebaceous glands

These tiny organs usually open into hair follicles on the surface of your skin. They produce an oily secretion, called sebum, which is your skin's natural lubricant.

The sebaceous glands are concentrated mostly on the scalp and face – particularly around the nose, cheeks, chin and forehead, which is why these are usually the most oily areas of your skin. The oily areas across the forehead and down the nose and chin are called the T-zone.

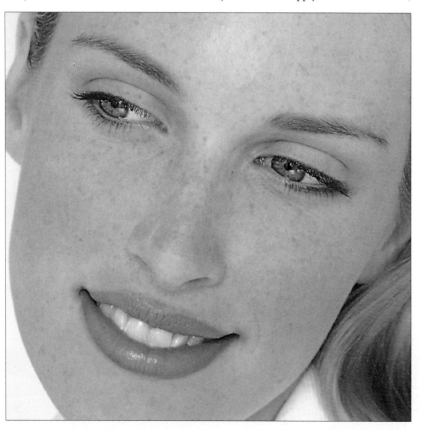

Left: Understanding your skin in the way a beautician would allows you to give it the care it deserves and to appreciate why certain factors are good for it – and others are not.

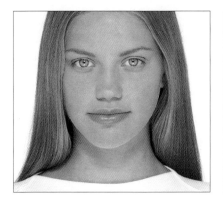

Above: Your skin is a sensor of pain, touch and temperature, offering protection to your inner body and a means of eliminating waste.

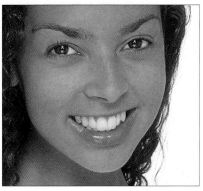

Above: Your skin can cleanse, heal and even renew itself. How effectively it does these things is partly governed by how you care for it.

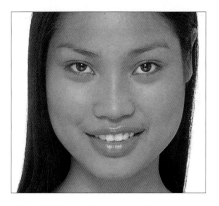

Above: Skin is a barometer of your emotions. It becomes red when you're embarrassed and quickly begins to show the signs of stress.

Sweat glands

There are millions of sweat glands all over your body, and their main function is to regulate your body temperature. When sweat evaporates on the skin's surface, the temperature of your skin drops.

Hairs

Hairs grow from hair follicles. They can help keep your body warm by trapping air underneath them.

THE MAIN FUNCTIONS OF YOUR SKIN

■ It acts as a thermostat, retaining heat or cooling you down with sweat.

■ It offers protection from potentially harmful things.

■ It acts as a waste disposal. Certain waste is expelled from your body 24 hours a day through your skin.

■ It provides you with a sense of touch.

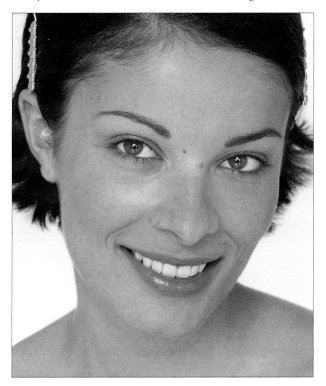

Left: The condition of your skin is an overall sign of your health. It reveals stress, a poor diet and a lack of sleep. Taking care of your health will benefit your skin.

Eating for a Beautiful Skin

While lotions and potions can improve your skin from the outside, a healthy diet works from the inside out. A nutritious, balanced diet isn't only a delicious way to eat – it can work wonders for your skin.

YOU ARE WHAT YOU EAT

A diet for a healthy body is the same one as for a healthy, clear complexion. That

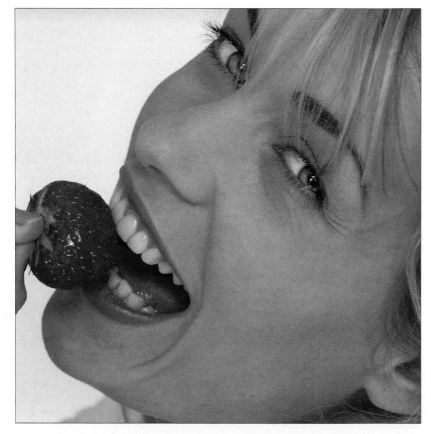

Above: A fresh and fruity diet will keep your complexion looking good.

is, one that contains lots of fresh fruit and vegetables, is high in fibre, low in fat, and low in added sugar and salt. This should provide your body and your skin with all the vitamins and minerals needed to function at their very best.

HEALTHY SKIN CHECKLIST

These are the essentials your body needs to keep your skin in tip-top condition.

1 The most essential element is water. Although there's water in the foods you eat, you should drink at least two litres (quarts) of water a day to keep your body healthy and your skin clear.

2 Cellulose carbohydrates, better known as fibre foods, have another less direct effect on your skin. Their action in keeping you regular can help to give you a brighter, clearer complexion.

3 Vitamin A is essential for growth and repair of certain skin tissues. Lack of it causes dryness, itching and loss of skin elasticity. It's found in foods such as carrots, spinach, broccoli and apricots.

4 Vitamin C is needed for collagen production, which helps keep your skin firm. It's found in foods such as strawberries, citrus fruits, cabbage, tomatoes and watercress.

5 Vitamin E is an antioxidant vitamin that neutralizes free radicals – highly reactive molecules that can cause ageing. It occurs in foods such as almonds, hazelnuts and wheat germ.

6 Zinc works with vitamin A in the making of collagen and elastin, the fibres that give your skin its strength, elasticity and firmness.

DIET Q & A

A healthy diet and beautiful complexion go hand in hand. Check to make sure you know the facts.

Q "Is it true that constantly losing and gaining weight can have a bad effect on your skin?"

A Yes. Eating too much and becoming overweight thickens the layer of fat under your skin and consequently stretches it. Crash dieting can then result in your skin collapsing, leading to the appearance of lines and wrinkles. What's more, a crash diet will deprive your skin and body of the essential nutrients they need to stay healthy and look good. If you need to lose weight, do it slowly, sensibly and steadily, to give your skin time to acclimatize (acclimate). It's always advisable to consult your doctor before starting any weight loss programme.

Q "What would be a good typical day's diet for a clearer complexion?"

A One that follows the rules already outlined. For example, here's a typical day you could follow.

Breakfast: A glass of unsweetened fruit juice; a bowl of unsweetened muesli (whole grain cereal), topped with a chopped banana and semi-skimmed (one per cent or skim) milk; two slices of whole wheat toast with a scraping of low-fat spread.

Lunch: Baked potato, filled with low-fat cottage cheese and plenty of fresh, raw salad; one low-fat yogurt, any flavour.

Evening meal: Grilled (broiled) fish or chicken, with boiled brown rice and plenty of steamed vegetables. Fresh fruit salad, topped with natural yogurt and nuts.

Q "Does chocolate cause pimples?"

A There isn't any scientific evidence that links eating chocolate to having break-outs, but as a healthy low-fat, high-fibre diet is known to be good for skin, keep snacks such as chocolate to a minimum and eat them only as an occasional treat.

Right: It's obvious that drinking plenty of water during the day helps purify your body – which means fresher, firmer skin.

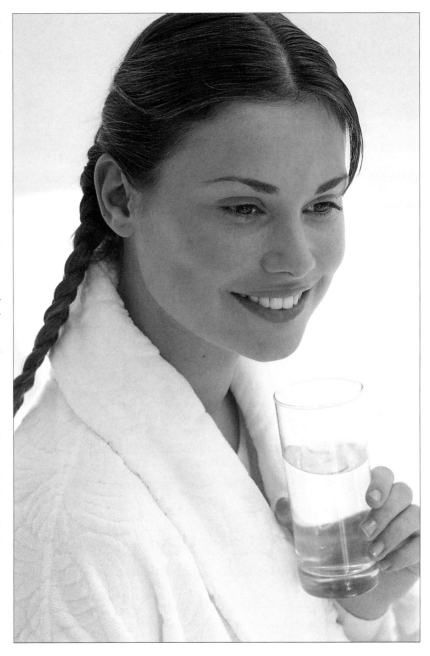

What's your Skin Type?

There's no point spending a fortune on expensive skincare products if you buy the wrong ones for your skin type. The key to developing a skincare regime that works for you is to analyze your skin type first.

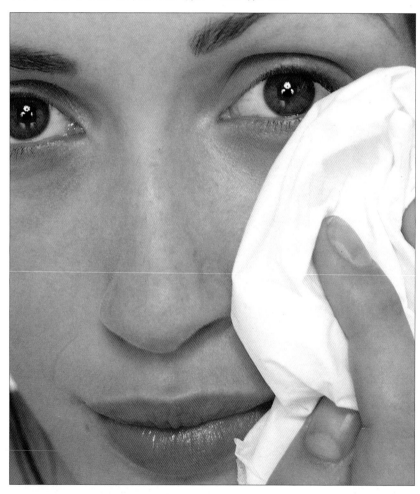

Above: You know best how your skin reacts to different things so check your skin type before you buy lots of skincare products. Even if you've been told what your skin type is at some stage, it is a good idea to run through this quiz now as your skin will change over a period of time.

SKINCARE QUIZ

To develop a better understanding of your skin and what skincare routine and products will suit it best, start by answering the questions here. Then add up your score and check the list at the end to discover which of the skin types you fit into. Remember that your skin type can change over time — try to do this skincare quiz each year to check that you are still using the right skincare products and following the best skincare routine.

1 How does your skin feel if you cleanse it with facial wash (soap) and water?
A Tight, as though it's too small for my face.
B Smooth and comfortable.
C Dry and itchy in places.
D Fine – quite comfortable.
E Dry in some areas and smooth in others.

2 How does your skin feel if you cleanse it with cream cleanser?
A Relatively comfortable.
B Smooth and comfortable.
C Sometimes comfortable, sometimes itchy.
D Quite oily.
E Oily in some areas and smooth in others.

3 How does your skin usually look by midday?
A Flaky patches appearing.
B Fresh and clean.
C Flaky patches and some redness.
D Shiny.
E Shiny in the T-zone.

4 How often do you break out in spots?

A Hardly ever.

B Occasionally, perhaps before or during your period.

C Occasionally.

D Often.

E Often – in the T-zone.

5 How does your skin react when you use facial toner?

A It stings.

B No problems.

C Stings and itches.

D Feels fresher.

E Feels fresher in some areas but stings in others.

6 How does your skin react to a rich night cream?

A It feels very comfortable.

B Comfortable.

C Sometimes feels comfortable, other times feels irritated.

D Makes my skin feel very oily.

E Oily in the T-zone, and comfortable on the cheeks.

Now add up the number of As, Bs, Cs, Ds and Es. Your skin type is the one which has the majority of answers. You are now ready to follow the right skincare routine for your skin type.

Mostly As: Your skin is DRY.

Mostly Bs: Your skin is NORMAL.

Mostly Cs: Your skin is SENSITIVE.

Mostly Ds: Your skin is OILY.

Mostly Es: Your skin is COMBINATION.

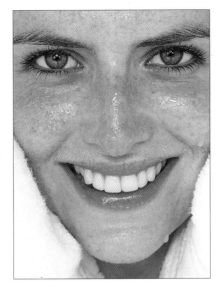

Above: Is traditional soap and water cleansing right for you?

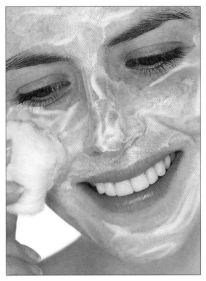

Above: Or is the gentle touch of a cleansing cream a softer option?

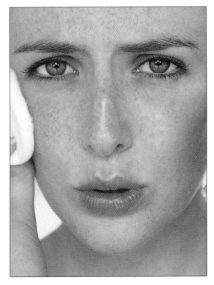

Above: Does using a facial toner make your skin sting?

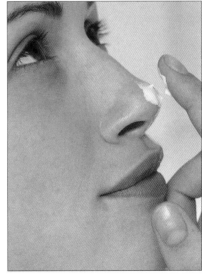

Above: Are your face creams an embarrassment of riches?

The Top Skincare Products

Before you can devise the best regime for yourself and give your skin some special care, you need to understand what the main skincare products are designed to do. From a basic soap and water cleansing routine, today's skincare ranges have evolved into a sophisticated selection.

Facial washes

These scrubs are designed to be lathered up with water to dissolve grime, dirt and stale make-up from the skin's surface.

Cleansing bars

A wash to cleanse your skin without stripping it of moisture – ordinary soap is too drying for most skins. They're refreshing for oilier skin types and help keep pores clear and prevent pimples.

Cream cleansers

These light creams are a wonderful way to cleanse drier complexions. They generally have quite a light, fluid consistency to make them easy to spread onto the skin. They contain oils to dissolve surface dirt and make-up, so they can be easily swept from your skin with cotton wool (cotton balls). Use damp cotton wool if you prefer a fresher finish.

Toners and astringents

Designed to refresh and cool your skin, toners quickly evaporate after being applied to the skin with cotton wool (cotton balls). They can also remove excess oil from the surface layers of your skin. The word "astringent" on the bottle means it has a higher alcohol content and is only suitable for oily skins. The words "tonic" and "toner" mean that they're useful for normal or combination skins, as they are gentler. Those with dry and sensitive skins should usually avoid these products, as they can be too drying. Generally, if the product stings your face, move onto a gentler formulation or weaken it by adding a few drops of distilled water (available from a pharmacist).

Moisturizers

These creams form a barrier film on the surface of your skin and prevent moisture loss from the top layers. This makes the skin feel softer and smoother. Generally, the drier your skin the thicker the moisturizer you should choose. All skin types need a moisturizer.

Moisturizers today also contain a myriad of other ingredients to treat your skin. The most valuable one to look for is an ultraviolet (UV) filter. With this, your moisturizer will give your skin year-round protection from the ageing and burning rays of the sun.

Eye make-up removers

When ordinary cleansers aren't sufficient to remove stubborn eye make-up, use a special make-up remover. If you wear waterproof mascara check that the product you use is designed to remove it.

Night creams

These are thick creams designed to give your skin extra moisturizing and pampering while you sleep.

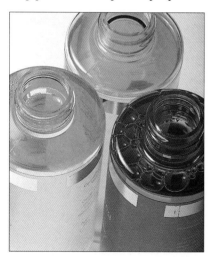

Above: Put some zing into your skincare regime with a refreshing toner or astringent treatment.

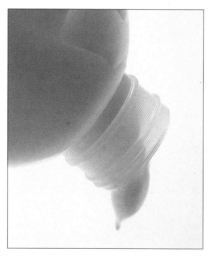

Above: Creamy cleansers should be a top priority for drier complexions, as they cleanse and nourish at the same time.

Right: Before you make up a skincare regime for yourself, you need to know the key benefits of each product.

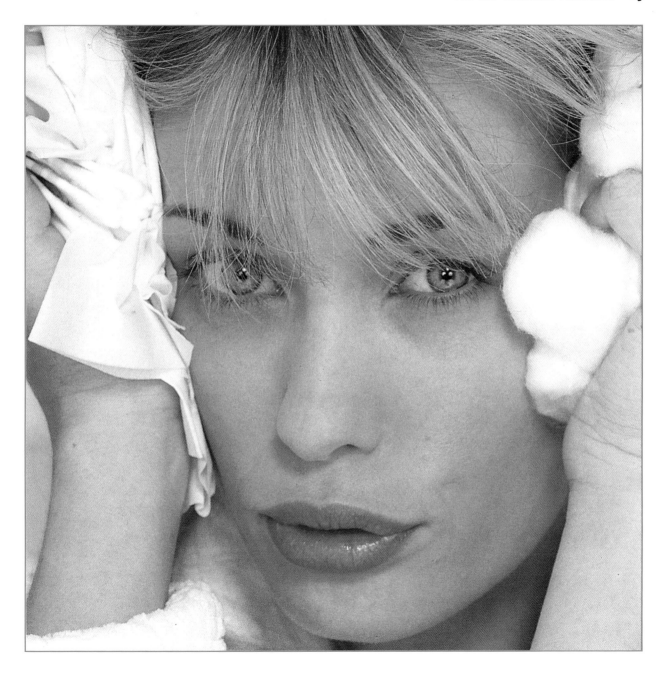

The Perfect Skincare Routine

Skincare can be confusing these days because there are so many products around. Basically, your skin needs two staples: cleanser and moisturizer. Other products – toner, exfoliator, and eye cream or gel – are extras. If you are using more than three or four products daily and your skin keeps breaking out or reacting, you may be trying too hard. Simplify your routine (it should not take more than 10 minutes to do twice a day), and use basic formulas. You really will be amazed by the speed at which your skin improves.

Cleanse

Use water-soluble emulsions (creams) or gels with tepid (not hot) water or wipe-off lotions. If your skin is oily, use pH-balanced soap-free bars. Splash your face with water – it will instantly give your skin a better tone.

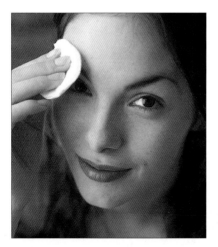

Above: Toners improve skin texture. Apply to oily skin after cleansing.

Tone

If you want to tone, buy alcohol-free toner or use rosewater to freshen your skin. If your skin is dry and you have been using toner, stop and it will instantly improve.

Moisturize

Ideally, use water-based creams and emulsions; if your skin frequently breaks out in pimples and blackheads, try a lighter, oil-free moisturizer.

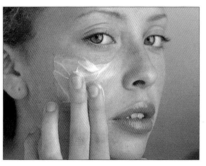

Above: Use upward and outward strokes to apply moisturizer.

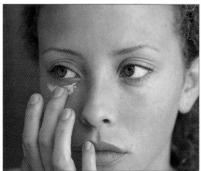

Above: Pat under-eye creams, gels and face creams on with your fingertips.

Exfoliate

Do this once a week only. Too much buffing will overstimulate and irritate your skin. Fine-grained exfoliators remove dead skin cells and instantly soften your skin.

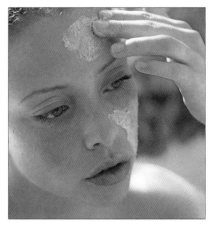

Above and below: Fine-grained exfoliators should be massaged gently into the skin and then rinsed away thoroughly.

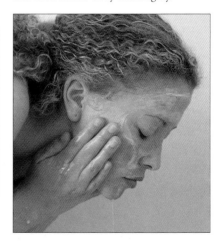

Mask

Simple mud- and clay-based cleansing masks are messy but effective. Rich cold creams make good moisturizing masks for dry or sun-exposed skin: smother your skin with the cream, let the skin absorb as much of the cream as possible and wipe off the excess with soft tissue.

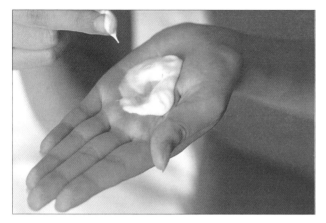

1 Put some of the mask into your hand first.

Then stroke it over clean, exfoliated skin, avoiding the eye area.

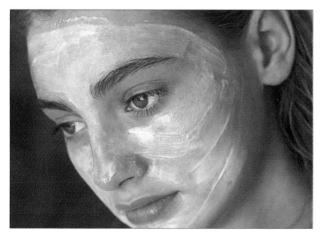

3 Relax for at least 10 minutes.

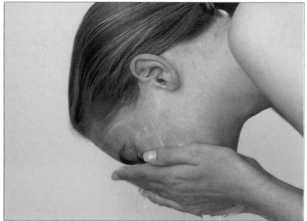

4 Rinse the face mask off thoroughly with tepid or warm water.

Maintaining Normal Skin

This is the perfect, balanced skin type. It has a healthy glow, with a fine texture and no open pores. It rarely develops spots or shiny areas. In fact, it's quite rare to find a normal skin, especially as all skins tend to become slightly drier as you get older.

SPECIAL CARE FOR NORMAL SKIN

Your main concern is to keep normal skin functioning well and, as a result of this, to let it continue the good job it's already doing. It naturally has a good balance of oil and moisture levels. Your routine should include gently cleansing your skin to ensure that surface grime and stale make-up are removed, and to prevent a build-up of sebum. Then you should boost moisture levels with moisturizer, to protect your skin and ensure its moisture content is balanced.

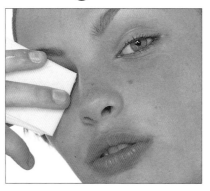

1 Eye make-up should always be removed carefully. Going to bed with mascara on can lead to sore, puffy eyes. Applying new make-up on the top of stale make-up is positively unhygienic too. Choose your product according to whether you're wearing ordinary or waterproof mascara.

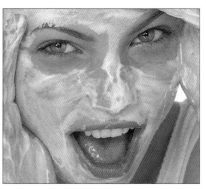

2 Splash your face with water, then massage in a gentle facial wash and work it up to a lather for about 30 seconds. Take this opportunity to lightly massage your face, as this will boost the supply of blood to the surface of your skin – which will result in a rosier complexion.

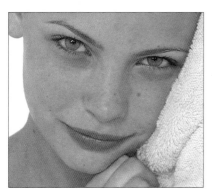

3 Rinse with clear water, then pat your face with a soft towel to absorb residual water from the surface of your skin. Don't rub at your skin, especially around the eyes, as this can encourage wrinkling.

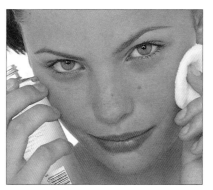

4 Cool your skin with a freshening toner. Again, be careful to avoid the delicate eye area as this can become more prone to dryness.

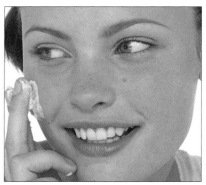

5 Dot moisturizer onto your face, then massage it in with your fingertips using light, gentle upward strokes. This will leave a protective film on the skin and allow make-up to be easily applied.

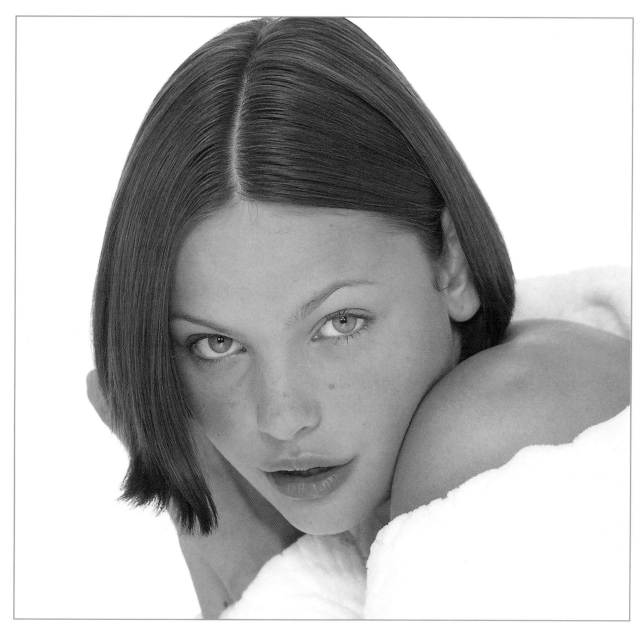

Above: Follow a regular skincare regime to keep normal skin as fresh as a daisy.

The Fresh Approach to Oily Skin

This skin type usually has open pores and an oily surface, with a tendency towards pimples, blackheads and a sallow appearance. This is due to the overproduction of sebum. Unfortunately, this skin type is the one most prone to acne. The good news is that this oiliness will make your skin stay younger-looking for longer – so there are some benefits!

SPECIAL CARE FOR OILY SKIN

It's important not to treat oily skin too harshly, although this can be tempting when you're faced with a fresh outbreak of pimples. Overenthusiastic treatment can encourage the oil glands to produce even more sebum, whilst it will leave the surface layers dry and dehydrated.

The best way to care for oily skin is to use products that gently cleanse away oils from the surface and unblock pores, without drying out and damaging it. The visible part of your skin actually needs water, not oil, to stay soft and supple.

ACNE ALERT

Anyone who has acne knows what a distressing condition it is. As well as being a problem that runs in families, it's thought to be triggered by a change in hormones during adolescence, which results in more sebum being produced by your skin. It can also be aggravated by stress, poor lifestyle and poor skincare.

Careful skincare will help keep acne under control. Avoid picking at pimples, as this can lead to scarring. Try over-the-counter blemish treatments. Today's formulations contain ingredients that are very successful at treating this problem. Products containing tea tree oil can be very effective. If these aren't successful, consult your doctor who may be able to provide treatment or refer you to a specialist dermatologist.

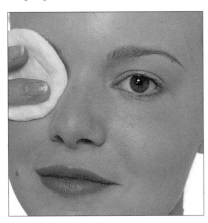

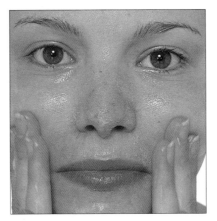

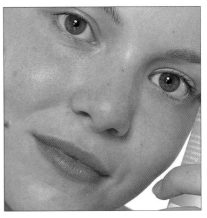

1 Even though the remainder of your face is prone to oiliness, always remember that the skin around your eyes is very delicate. Soak a cotton wool (cotton ball) pad with a non-oily remover and hold it over your eyes for a few seconds to give it time to dissolve the make-up. Then lightly stroke away the mascara and make-up from the eyelids and your upper and lower lashes.

2 Splash your face with tepid water, then lather up with a gentle foaming facial wash. This is a better choice than ordinary soap, as it won't strip away moisture from your skin, but it will remove the grime, dirt and oil that accumulates during the day. Massage gently over damp skin with your fingertips, then carefully rinse away with lots of warm water.

3 Soak a cotton wool (cotton ball) pad with a refreshing astringent lotion. Sweep it over your skin to refresh and cool it. This liquid should not irritate or sting your skin – if it does, swap to a product with a gentler formulation or dilute your existing one with some distilled water (available from a pharmacist). Continue until the cotton wool comes up completely clean.

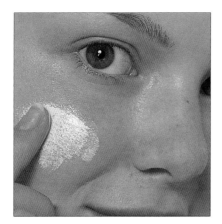

4 Even oily skin needs a gentle moisturizer, because a moisturizer helps to seal water into the top layers of the skin to keep your face soft and supple. Choose a light, watery fluid rather than a heavy formulation, as this will be enough for you.

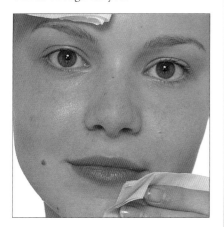

5 Allow the moisturizer to sink into your skin for a few minutes, then press a clean tissue over your face to absorb the excess and to prevent a shiny complexion.

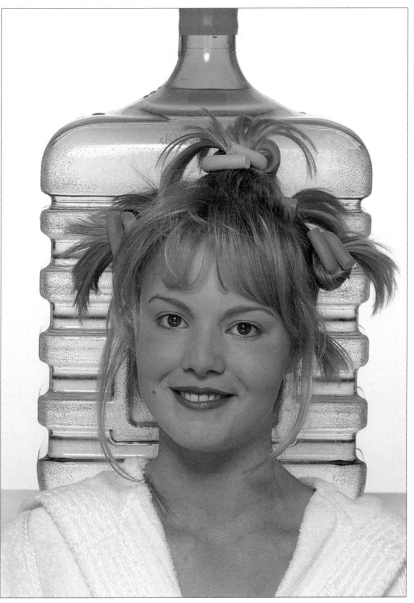

Above: Boosting your skin's moisture levels and controlling excess oiliness will ensure a beautifully clear complexion.

Nourishing Care for Dry Skin

If your skin tends to feel one size too small, it's a fair bet you've got a dry complexion. It's caused by too little sebum in the lower levels of the skin and too little moisture in the upper levels. It can feel tight after washing. At its worst, it can be flaky, with flakiness in your eyebrows, and have a tendency to promote premature ageing with the emergence of fine lines and wrinkles.

SPECIAL CARE FOR DRY SKIN

The condition of dry skin can be aggravated by overuse of soap, detergents and toners. It is also affected by exposure to hot sun, cold winds and central heating. Opt for the gentle approach, concentrating on boosting the skin's moisture level to plump out fine lines and make it soft and supple.

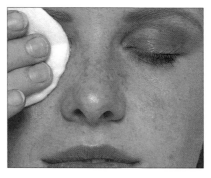

1 Pour a little oil-based eye make-up remover onto a cotton wool (cotton ball) pad and sweep it over the eye area. This oily product will also help soothe dryness in the delicate eye area, but a little goes a long way. If you overload the skin here with an oily product it can cause puffiness and irritation.

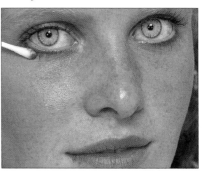

2 Clean up stubborn flecks with a cotton bud (swab) dipped in eye make-up remover. Be careful not to get the remover in your eyes but work as closely as you can to the eyelashes to remove all signs of make-up.

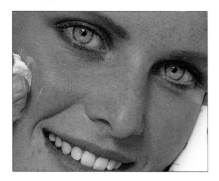

3 Choose a creamy cleanser that will melt away dirt and make-up from the surface of your skin. Leave the cleanser on for a few moments for it to work, before sweeping it away with a cotton wool (cotton ball) pad. Use gentle upward movements to prevent stretching the skin and encouraging lines.

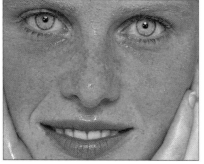

4 Many women with dry skins say that they miss the feeling of water on their skin. However, you can splash your face with cool water to remove excess cleanser and to refresh your skin. This will also help boost the blood circulation in your face, which means a brighter complexion.

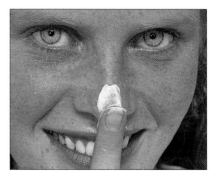

5 This is the most important step of all for dry skins – a nourishing cream to seal moisture into the upper levels of your skin. Opt for a thick cream, rather than a runny lotion, as this contains more oil than water. Give the moisturizer a few minutes to sink into your skin before applying make-up.

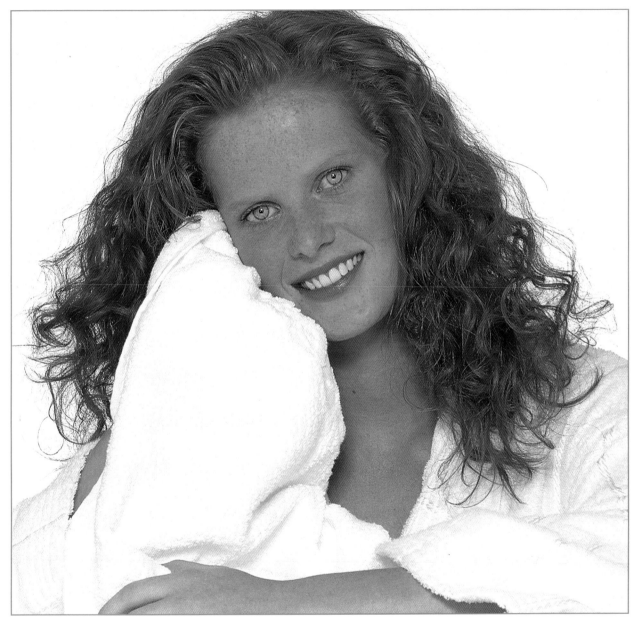

Above: Nourish dry skin by using a thick moisturizer to keep it as soft and supple as possible.

Balanced Care for Combination Skin

Combination skin needs careful attention because it has a blend of oily and dry patches. The centre panel, or T-zone, across the forehead and down the nose and chin tends to be oily and needs to be treated like oily skin. However, the other areas are prone to dryness and flakiness due to lack of moisture and need to be treated like dry skin. Having said this, some combination skins don't follow the T-zone pattern and can have patches of dry and oily skin in other arrangements. If you're unsure of your skin's oily and dry areas, press a tissue to your face an hour after washing it. Any greasy patches on the tissue signify oily areas — this will enable you to develop a routine appropriate for your skin.

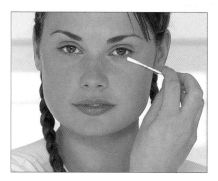

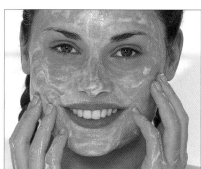

1 Choose an oil-based eye make-up remover to clear away every trace of eye make-up from this delicate area, which is prone to dryness. Use a cotton bud (swab) to remove any stubborn traces. Splash with cool water afterwards to rinse away any excess oil.

2 Use a foaming facial wash in the morning to cleanse your skin. This will ensure the oily areas are clean and that the pores on your nose are kept clear. Massage a little onto damp skin, concentrating on the oily areas. Leave for a few seconds to dissolve the dirt, then rinse.

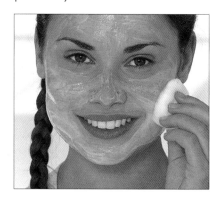

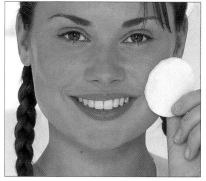

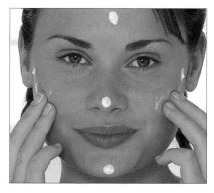

3 In the evening, switch to a cream cleanser, to ensure the dry areas of your skin are kept clean and soothed on a daily basis. This will give you a balance between excess oiliness or dryness. Massage well into your skin, concentrating on the drier areas, then remove with cotton wool pads (cotton balls).

4 To freshen your skin, you need to use two different strengths of toners. Choose a stronger astringent for the oily areas, and a mild skin freshener for the drier ones. This isn't as expensive as you think, because you'll only need to use a little of each. Sweep over your skin with cotton wool pads (cotton balls).

5 Smooth moisturizer onto your entire skin, concentrating on the drier areas. Then blot off any excess from the oily areas with a tissue.

Right: A twin approach to skincare will double the benefits for combination skin, and it needn't be time consuming.

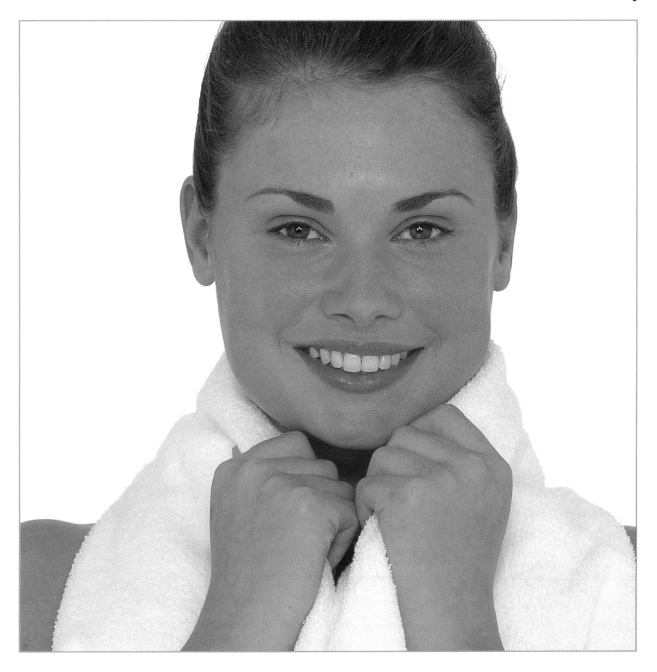

Soothing Care for Sensitive Skin

Sensitive skin is usually quite fine in texture, with a tendency to be rosier than usual. Easily irritated by products and external factors, it's also prone to redness and allergy and may have fine broken veins across the cheeks and nose. There are varying levels of sensitivity. If you feel you can't use any products on your skin without irritating it, cleanse with whole milk and moisturize with a solution of glycerin and rosewater. These should soothe it.

CARING FOR SENSITIVE SKIN

Your skin needs extra-gentle products to keep it healthy. Choose from hypoallergenic ranges that are specially formulated to protect sensitive skin. They're screened for common irritants, such as fragrance, that can cause dryness, itchiness or even an allergic reaction. Remember to moisturize your skin well as dryness can make sensitive skin even more uncomfortable. Don't forget to choose an unperfumed moisturizer.

> **Tip**
> If you have particularly sensitive skin, try using an evening primrose oil moisturizer. It's a wonderful natural moisturizer, particularly for dry or very dry skins, as it hydrates, protects and soothes. It also improves the skin's overall softness and suppleness. Many sufferers of eczema also find it useful.

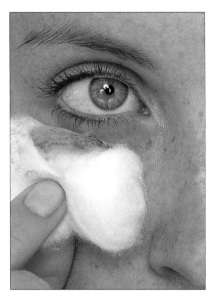

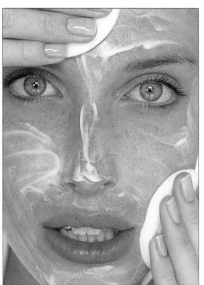

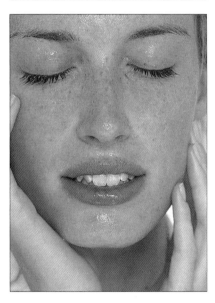

1 Make sure that the make-up you use is hypoallergenic, too, and remove it thoroughly. First use a soothing eye make-up remover. Apply with a cotton wool (cotton ball) pad, then remove every last trace with a clean cotton bud (swab).

2 Avoid facial washes and soaps on your skin, as these are likely to strip the skin of oil and moisture, which can increase your skin's sensitivity even more. So, instead, choose a light, hypoallergenic cleansing lotion.

3 Even the mildest skin freshener can break down the natural protection your delicate skin needs against the elements. So freshen it by simply splashing with warm water instead. This will also remove the final traces of cleanser and eye make-up remover from your skin.

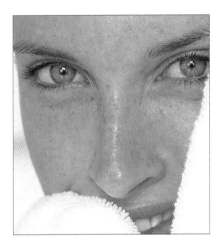

4 Lightly pat your face dry with a soft towel, taking care not to rub the skin as this could irritate it.

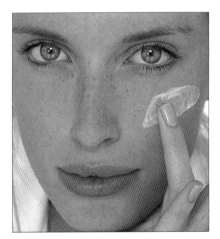

5 It's essential to keep your skin well moisturized to strengthen it and provide a barrier against irritants that can lead to sensitivity.

Right: Careful skincare will take the sting out of sensitive skins.

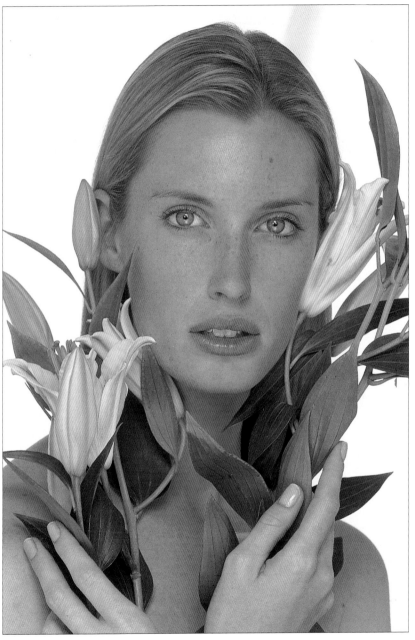

Try a Fabulous Facial

For deep-down cleansing and a definite improvement in skin tone, try an at-home facial. Just once a month will make a noticeable difference to your complexion. Follow these steps to re-create the benefits of the beauty salon in the comfort and privacy of your own home.

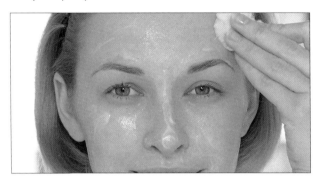

1 Smooth your skin with cleansing cream. Leave on for 1-2 minutes to give it time to dissolve grime, oils and stale make-up. Then gently smooth away excess cream with cotton wool pads (cotton balls).

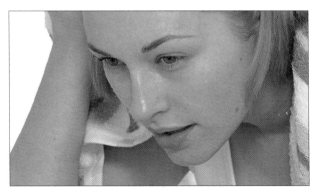

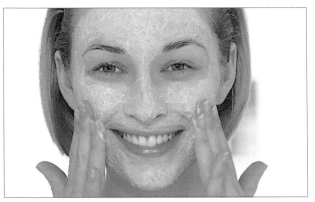

2 Dampen your skin with warm water, then gently massage in a blob of facial scrub using your fingertips, avoiding the delicate eye area. This will loosen dead surface skin cells and leave your skin softer and smoother. It will also prepare your complexion for the beneficial treatments to come. Rinse with warm water.

3 Fill a wash basin (sink) with boiling water. Lean over the top, capturing the steam with a towel draped over your head. Stay there for five minutes and then gently remove any blackheads with tissue-covered fingers. If you have sensitive skin, or broken veins, you should avoid this step.

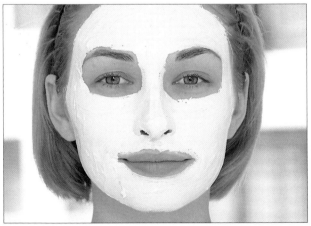

4 Smooth on a face mask. Choose a clay-based one if you have oily skin, or a moisturizing one if you have dry or normal skin. Leave on for five minutes, or for as long as specified by the instructions on the product.

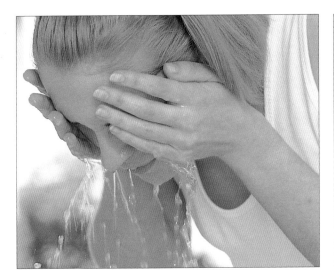

5 Rinse away the face mask with warm water. Finish off with a few splashes of cool water to close your pores and freshen your skin, then pat dry with a towel.

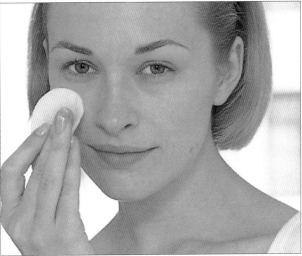

6 Soak a cotton wool (cotton ball) pad with a skin toner lotion and smooth over oily areas, such as the T-zone on the nose, chin and forehead.

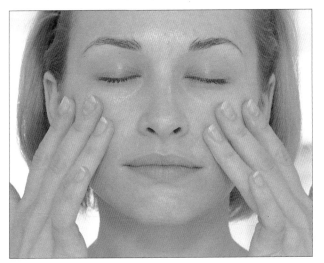

7 Dot your skin with moisturizer and smooth it in. Take the opportunity to massage your skin, as this encourages a brighter complexion and can help reduce puffiness.

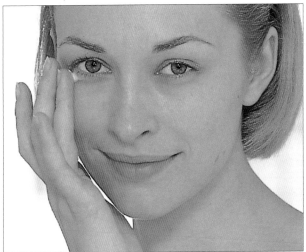

8 Smooth the senstive area under your eyes with a soothing eye cream to reduce fine lines and wrinkles, and make the skin ultrasoft.

Delicate Care for Eyes

The fine skin around the eyes is the first to show the signs of ageing, as well as dark circles and puffiness. It needs extra special care because it's thinner than the skin on the rest of your face, so it's less able to hold in moisture. There are also fewer oil glands in this area, which adds to the potential dryness, and there's no fatty layer underneath the skin to act as a shock absorber. The result is that this skin quickly loses it elasticity.

CHOOSING AN EYE TREATMENT

Face creams and oils are too heavy for the eye area. They can block tear ducts, causing puffiness, so you should choose a specific eye treatment that won't aggravate your skin. There are hundreds of products to choose from. Gel-based ones are great for young or oily skins and are refreshing to use. However, most women find light eye creams and balms are gentler and more suitable.

Apply a tiny amount of the eye treatment with your ring finger, as this is the weakest one on your hand. It's better to apply it regularly in small quantities than to apply lots only occasionally. This will help keep your skin more supple and prevent premature wrinkling in this area.

Right: Try placing cucumber slices over the eyelids – they are a natural aid for puffy eyes.

Far right: Cotton wool pads (cotton balls) soaked in rosewater and put over the eyelids soothe tired eyes.

DE-PUFFING EYES

This is one of the most common beauty problems. These ideas can help:

■ Gently tap your skin with your ring finger when you're applying eye cream to encourage the excess fluid to drain away.

■ Store creams in the refrigerator, as the coldness will also help reduce puffiness.

■ Take a couple of slices of cucumber (or strips of grated potato) and rest them on your eyes for 20 minutes.

■ Rest for about 15 minutes with two damp tea bags over your eyes; tea bags are said to help fade under-eye bags because they contain tannin and polyphenols which have an astringent effect.

■ Fill a small bowl with iced water or ice-cold milk. Soak a cotton wool (cotton ball) pad with the liquid and lie down with the dampened pads over your eyes. Replace the pads as soon as they become warm. Continue for 15 minutes. As well as reducing puffiness, this treatment will brighten the whites of your eyes.

■ Soak two cotton wool wedges (cotton balls) in chilled rosewater, squeeze out the excess and rest them on your eyes for 20 minutes.

■ Leave a teaspoon in the fridge for an hour or overnight, remove it and place the bulb of the spoon over your eye, first making sure it is not too cold or freezing, as this may damage your skin.

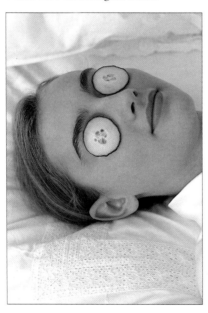

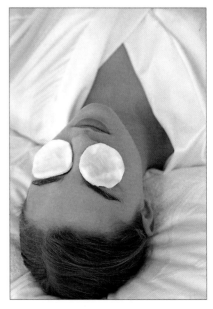

Good Night Creams

Going to bed with night cream on your face can benefit your skin while you sleep. Your skin's cell renewal is more active during the night, and night creams are designed to make the most of these hours. Using a night cream gives your skin the chance to repair the daily wear and tear caused by pollution, make-up and ultraviolet light.

What are night creams?

The main difference between night creams and ordinary daily moisturizers is that most night creams have added ingredients such as vitamins and anti-ageing components. They can be thicker and more intensive than day creams because you don't need to wear make-up on top of them.

Who needs night creams?

While very young skins don't really need the extra nourishing properties of night creams, most women find that they benefit from using one. Dry and very dry skins respond particularly well. You don't have to choose very rich formulations, as there are now lighter alternatives that contain the same special ingredients. Choose the best formulation on the basis of how dry your skin is – it shouldn't feel overloaded.

> **Tip**
> Applying night cream to slightly damp skin can really boost its performance, as this helps to seal in extra moisture – which means softer and smoother skin the next morning.

Below left: Applying night cream just before you go to bed means waking up to a softer complexion.

Below: Dry areas, like cheeks, will absorb the extra moisture a rich night cream can provide.

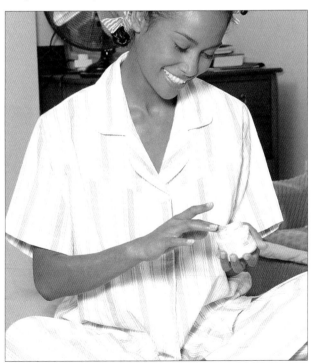

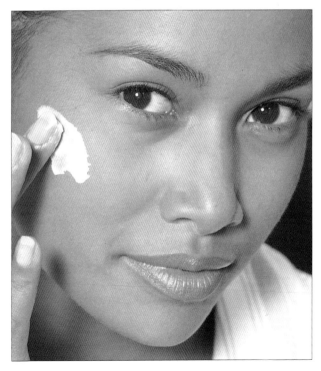

Miraculous Masks

If there's one skincare item that can work immediate miracles, it's a face mask. But, like any other skincare product, you can't just reach for the first one and hope for the best. You should choose carefully to pick the perfect product for you.

MASK IT!

Choose from the wonderful selection of face masks on the market.

Moisturizing masks

Suitable for dry complexions, these rich masks will boost the moisture levels of your skin. This means they can help banish dry patches, flakiness and even fine lines. They work quickly like an intensive moisturizer and are usually left on the skin for 5-10 minutes before being removed with tissue. The slight residue left on the skin will continue to work until it is next cleansed. They're a great treat, particularly after sunbathing, or when your skin feels "tight".

Clay and mud masks

Oily skins need a clay or mud mask to absorb excess grease and impurities from the skin. They're an ideal way to "shrink" open pores, blot out shininess and clear away troublesome blemishes. They dry on your skin over a period of 5-15 minutes, then you simply wash them away with warm water, rinsing dead skin cells, dirt and grime away at the same time. They're a great pick-me-up for skin.

Exfoliating masks

These deep-cleansing masks keep your skin in tip-top condition. Even normal skins sometimes suffer from the build-up of dead skin cells, which can create a dull look and lead to future problems, such as blackheads. Masks that cleanse and exfoliate are the perfect solution. They smooth on like a clay mask and are left to dry. When you rinse them away, their tiny abrasive particles wash away the skin's surface debris.

Peel-off masks

Try this technique; it's great for all skin types and fun to use. You smooth on the gel, leave it to dry, then peel it away. The light formulation will help refresh oily areas by clearing clogged pores, as well as lightly nourishing drier skins.

Gel masks

Gel masks are suitable for sensitive skins, as well as oily complexions, as they have a wonderfully soothing and cooling effect. You simply apply the gel, lie back and relax, then after 5-10 minutes remove the excess with tissue. They're wonderful after too much sun, or when your skin feels irritated.

Below: Clay and mud masks dry on your skin over a period of 5-15 minutes.

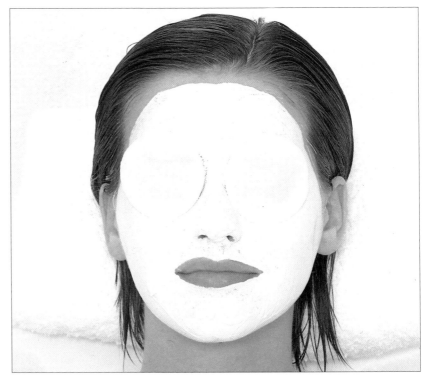

Facial Scrubs

Brighten up your complexion in an instant with this skincare treat. If you don't include a facial scrub in your weekly skincare regime, then you've been missing out. Technically known as exfoliation, it's a simple method that removes dead surface cells from the top of your skin, revealing the plumper, younger ones underneath. It also encourages your skin to speed up cell production, which means that the cells that reach the surface are younger and better looking. The result is a brighter, smoother complexion – no matter what your age.

ACTION TACTICS

Use an exfoliator on dry or normal skin once a week. Oily or combination skins can be exfoliated once or twice a week. As a rule, avoid this treatment on sensitive skin, or if you have bad acne. However, you can gently exfoliate pimple-prone skin once a week to help keep pores clear and to prevent breakouts.

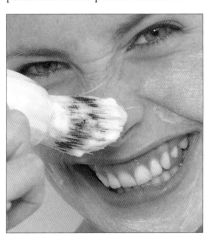

GETTING TO THE NITTY-GRITTY

■ Apply a blob of facial scrub cream to damp skin, massage gently, then rinse away with lots of cool water. Opt for an exfoliator that contains gentler, rounded beads, rather than scratchy ones like crushed kernels.

■ Try a mini exfoliating pad, lathering up with soap or facial wash.

Below: Get your skin glowing with a quick and easy facial treat.

Tip
Whichever method of exfoliation you choose to use, avoid scrubbing the delicate area around the eyes. This is because the skin is very fine here and it can easily be irritated.

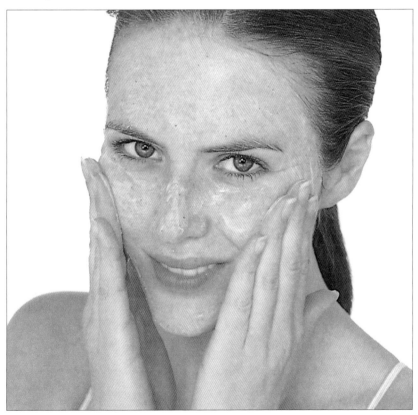

Left: Instead of using a facial scrub, gently massage your skin with a soft flannel (wash cloth), facial brush, or old, clean shaving brush.

Be a Fruity Beauty

Incorporated in small amounts, alpha-hydroxy acids (AHAs) have recently become a key ingredient in specialized skincare products. They've become the biggest skincare invention of the 1990s, and their success looks set to continue for many years. Many women find AHAs dramatically improve the condition and look of their skin.

AHA KNOW-HOW

Alpha-hydroxy acids, also commonly known as fruit acids, are found in natural products. These include citric acid from citrus fruit, lactic acid from sour milk, tartaric acid from wine, and malic acid from apples and other fruits.

AHAs work by breaking down the protein bonds that hold together the dead cells on the surface of your skin. They then lift them away and reveal the brighter, plumper cells underneath. This gentle process cleans and clears blocked pores, improves your skin tone and softens the look of fine lines. You should start to see results within a couple of weeks, although many women report that they see an improvement after only a few days.

Without even realizing the exact reasons for their improved skin, women have used AHAs for centuries. For example, Cleopatra is said to have bathed in sour asses' milk, and ladies of the French court applied wine to their faces to keep their skin smooth, supple and blemish free – both these ancient beauty aids are now known to contain AHAs.

AHA products are best used under your ordinary everyday moisturizer as a treatment cream. You should avoid applying them to the delicate eye and lip areas. If you have very sensitive skin, you may find they're not suitable for you, but some women experience a slight tingling sensation at first anyway, as the product gets to work.

The great news is that AHA products are now becoming more affordable, and not just the preserve of more expensive skincare companies. Many mid-market companies are including the benefits of AHAs in their products, so everyone can give their skin the high tech treatment it deserves. You can also find AHA products for the hands and body, so you can reap the benefits from head to toe.

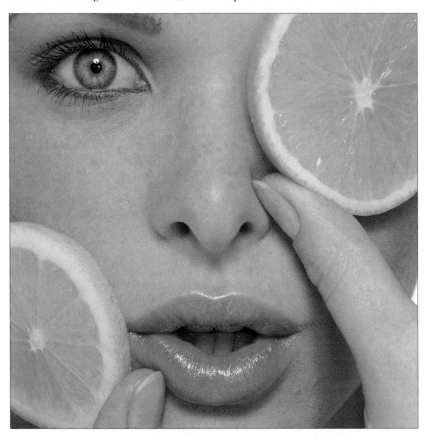

Above: AHAs (otherwise known as fruit acids) are an effective way to put the zing back into your skin. In fact, there's nothing new about AHAs – by bathing in asses' milk Cleopatra was absorbing AHAs into her skin.

Special Skin Treatments

You'd be forgiven for thinking you might need a PhD in chemistry to choose a skin treatment these days! As well as basic moisturizers, there are a whole host of special treatments, serums and gels that are designed to treat specific problems.

THE KEY TREATMENTS

You'll find that special skin treatments come in all shapes and sizes and in various formulations.

Serums and gels

These products have an ultra-light formulation, a non-greasy texture and a high concentration of active ingredients. They're not usually designed to be used on their own, except on oily skins. They're generally applied under a moisturizer to enhance its benefits and boost the anti-ageing process.

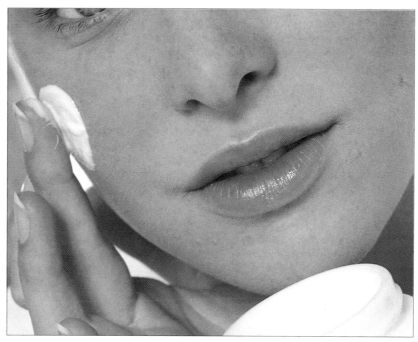

Above: Choose a cream that contains specialized ingredients to improve your skin.

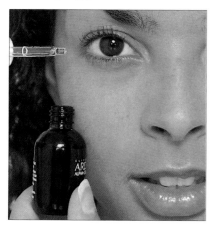

Above: Try using a few drops of special skin serum — it will work wonders for your skin.

Skin firmers

These creams are designed to tighten, firm and smooth your skin. They work by forming an ultra-fine film on the skin, which tightens your complexion and reduces the appearance of fine lines. The effects last for a few hours, and make-up can easily be applied on top. These products are a wonderful treat for a special night out or when you're feeling particularly tired.

Skin energizers

Speed up the natural production and repair of your skin cells with these creams that contain special ingredients. As well as producing a fresher, younger-looking skin, skin energizers are also thought to help combat the signs of ageing.

Ampule treatments

These special treatments are very concentrated active ingredients contained in sealed glass phials or ampules, to ensure that they're completely fresh. Typical extracts include herbs, wheat germ, vitamins and collagen – used for their intensive and fast-acting results. Vitamin E is another great, natural skin saver and healer. Break open a capsule and smooth the oil onto your face for an immediate skin treat.

10 Ways to Beat Wrinkles

Fine lines and wrinkles aren't inevitable. In fact, skin experts believe that most skin damage can be prevented with a little know-how and some special care. Here are the 10 main points to bear in mind, no matter what your age.

1 Protect your skin from the sun

The single biggest cause of skin ageing is sunlight. You should use a sunscreen every single day of the year. This will help prevent your skin from becoming prematurely aged, as well as guard against burning and of course the risk of skin cancer. The ageing rays of the sun are as prevalent in the cold winter months as in the hot summer ones, so it's a daily safeguard you should take.

2 Stop smoking

Cigarette smoke speeds up the ageing process because it strips your skin of oxygen and slows down the rate at which new cells are regenerated. It's responsible for giving the skin a grey, sluggish look, and it can also cause fine lines around the mouth because heavy smokers tend to be constantly pursing their lips to draw on a cigarette.

3 Deep cleanse

It's essential to ensure that your skin is clear of dead skin cells, dirt and make-up to give it a youthful, fresh glow. You don't have to use harsh products to do this – a creamy cleanser removed with cotton wool (cotton balls) is a good option for most women. If your skin is very dry, try massaging it with an oily cleanser. Leave it on your skin for a few minutes, then rinse away the excess with warm water.

4 Deep moisturize

You can either use a nourishing face mask, or apply a thick layer of your usual moisturizer or night cream to boost the water levels of your skin on a weekly basis. Whichever you choose, leave it on the skin for 5-10 minutes, then remove the excess with tissues. Apply to damp skin for greater effect.

5 Boost the circulation

Buy a gentle facial scrub or exfoliator, and use once a week to keep the surface of your skin soft and smooth. This will

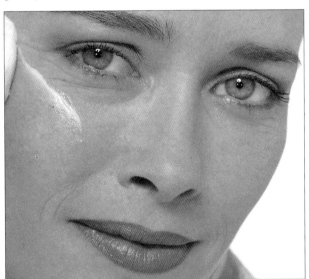

Above: You won't believe the difference regular cleansing can make to your skin.

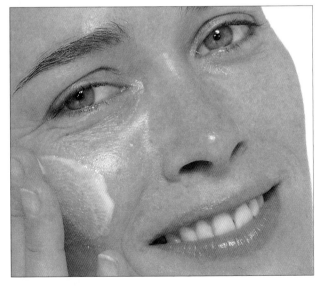

Above: Protect and survive by using a good moisturizer on a regular basis.

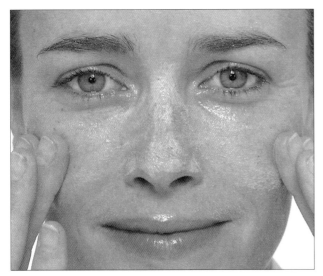

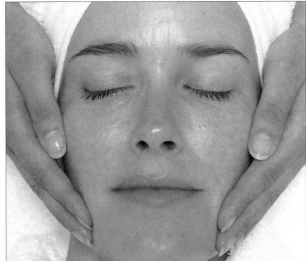

also increase the blood flow to the top layers of the skin, giving it a rosy glow and helping to encourage cell renewal. Alternatively, you can get the same effect by lathering up a facial wash on your skin using a clean shaving brush.

6 Disguise lines

Existing lines can be minimized to the naked eye by opting for the latest light-reflecting foundations, concealers and powders. These contain luminescent particles that bounce light away from your skin, making lines less noticeable and giving your skin a wonderful fresh-faced luminosity.

7 Pamper regularly

As well as a regular skincare regime, remember to treat your skin occasionally to special treatments such as facials, serums and anti-ageing creams. As well as improving the look of your skin, they'll encourage you to give it extra care on a regular basis.

8 Be weather vain

Extremes of cold and hot weather can strip your skin of essential moisture, leaving it dry and more prone to damage. Central heating can have the same effect. For this reason, ensure that you moisturize regularly, changing your products according to the seasons.

For instance, you may need a more oily product in the winter that will keep the cold out and won't freeze on the skin's surface. In hot weather, lighter formulations are more comfortable on the skin, and you can boost their activity by using a few drops of special treatment serum underneath.

9 Be gentle

Be careful you don't drag at your skin when applying skincare products or make-up. The skin around your eyes is particularly vulnerable. So, make sure you always use a light touch, and whenever you can, use upward and outward strokes, rather than dragging the

Above left: Wake up to the benefits of special skincare treatments.
Above: Relax and enjoy a beneficial facial - you'll reap the rewards.

skin down. When applying under-eye skin products, tap the cream on gently with the tip of your ring finger. Also, be careful to avoid any products that make your skin itch, sting or feel sensitive. If any product causes this sort of reaction, stop using it at once, and switch to a gentler formulation.

10 Clever make-up

Skincare benefits aren't just confined to skincare products these days. so investigate some of the latest make-up on offer. In fact, many make-up products now contain ultraviolet (UV) filters and skin-nourishing ingredients to treat your s kin as well as superficially improve its appearance. So investigate the latest products – it's well worth making use of them for 24-hour-a-day benefits.

How Well do you Care for your Body?

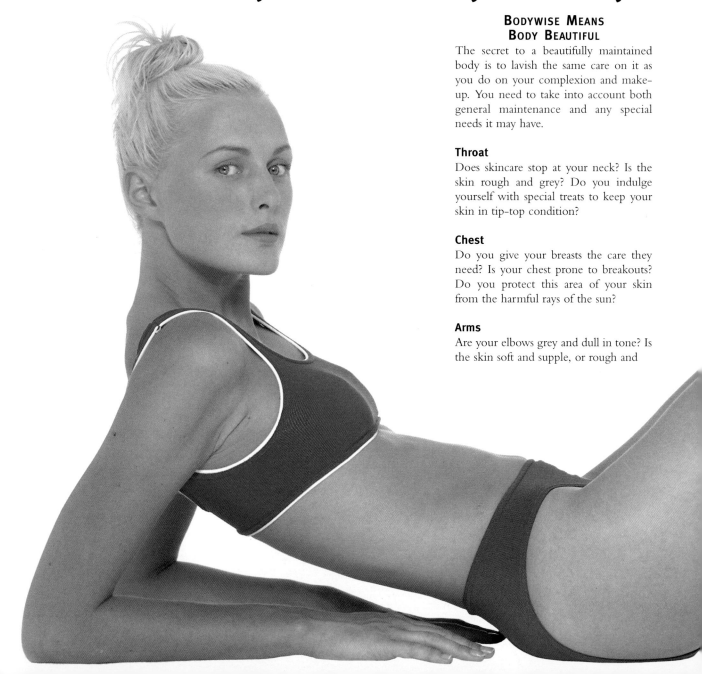

BODYWISE MEANS BODY BEAUTIFUL

The secret to a beautifully maintained body is to lavish the same care on it as you do on your complexion and make-up. You need to take into account both general maintenance and any special needs it may have.

Throat

Does skincare stop at your neck? Is the skin rough and grey? Do you indulge yourself with special treats to keep your skin in tip-top condition?

Chest

Do you give your breasts the care they need? Is your chest prone to breakouts? Do you protect this area of your skin from the harmful rays of the sun?

Arms

Are your elbows grey and dull in tone? Is the skin soft and supple, or rough and dry? Do darker hairs on your lower arms need bleaching? If you remove hair from your underarms, have you found the best method, the one that suits you for both convenience and results? Have you found the solution to underarm freshness?

Hands

Do your hands need moisturizing care? Are your nails neatly filed and shaped? Would a lick of polish or a French manicure give them a helping hand? Do you need to stop biting your nails?

Legs

Are your legs free from stubbly hair? Is the skin as smooth as it could be? Would they benefit from a light touch of fake tan? Are they prone to cellulite? Would bath time treats improve the look and feel of your skin?

Bikini line

If you remove hair from this area, have you found the best method for you?

Feet

Are your feet free from hard skin, corns and calluses? Are your nails neatly trimmed? Do you smooth a foot cream on them regularly to ensure that the skin stays soft?

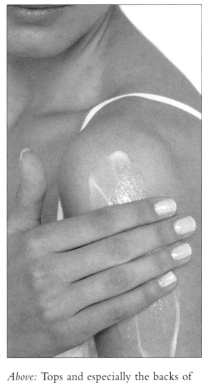

Above: Tops and especially the backs of arms need care too, so that they stay soft, supple and firm.

Bathroom Essentials

Caring for your body creates endless rewards. So, keep a selection of beauty products on hand to maintain your skin from head to toe on a daily and occasional basis.

BATHING BEAUTY

The time of day and even the time of year will affect what you like using, so why not take the opportunity to try different products, adding the ones you particularly like to those you already know well and use frequently.

Soaps and cleansing bars

These are a cheap and effective way of cleansing your body. If you find them too drying, choose ones that contain moisturizers to minimize these effects. Most people can use ordinary soaps and cleansers without any problem. However, if you have particularly dry or sensitive skin, opt for the pH-balanced variety.

Shower gels and bubble baths

Gels and bubbles provide mild detergents that cleanse your body while you soak in the water. There are hundreds of varieties to choose from, including those containing a host of additives, ranging from herbs to essential oils. If you find them too harsh for your skin, look for the ones that offer 2-in-1 benefits – these contain moisturizers as well, to soothe your skin.

Sponges and washcloths

Dislodge dirt and grime with a sponge or washcloth. They are also useful for lathering up soaps and gels on your skin. Wash your washcloth regularly, and allow it to dry between uses. Natural sponges are a more expensive but long-lasting alternative. Squeeze out afterwards in warm clear water and allow to dry naturally. However, don't underestimate the power of your hands for washing yourself; they keep you in touch with your body and will make you aware of any lumps, bumps and changes in texture that might occur.

Below: Wonder bars for the body.

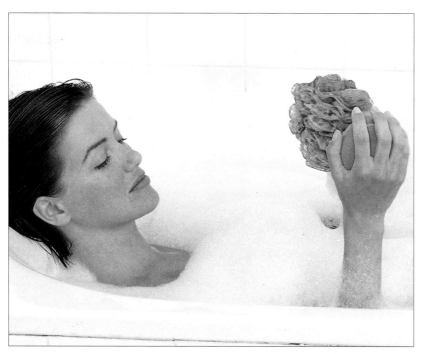

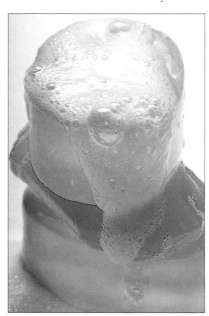

Left: Bubbles, bubbles – soothe away toils and troubles!

Bath oils

Oils for the bath are a wonderful beauty boon for those with dry skins. They float on the top of the water, and your entire body becomes covered with a fine film when you step out of the bath. Most cosmetic houses produce a bath oil, but if you're not worried about the fragrance, you can use a few drops of any vegetable oil, such as olive, corn or peanut.

Bath salts

Special salts made from sodium carbonate are particularly useful for softening hard water and for preventing your skin from becoming too dry. Combined with warm water, they're a popular way to soothe away aches and pains.

Below: Stock your bathroom shelves for head-to-toe freshness.

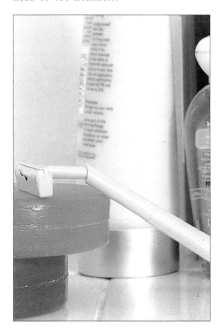

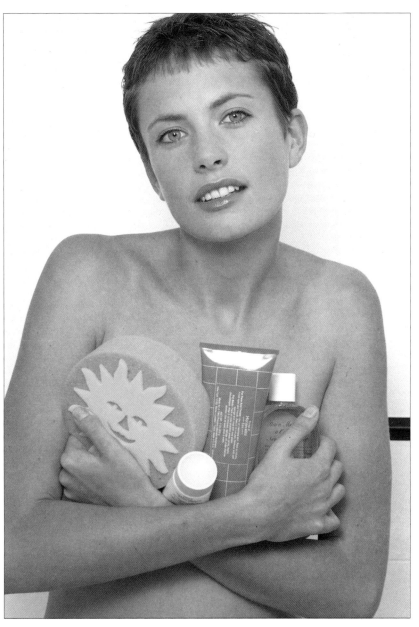

Above: Grab yourself some bathroom benefits.

Bathroom Treatments

As well as a chance to cleanse your body, bath or shower time is the perfect opportunity to pamper and polish your skin, and indulge in some beauty treats. Try some of these effective body treats on a regular basis.

Body lotions and oils

Seal moisture into your skin with a lotion or oil, making it soft and smooth. Especially concentrate on drier areas, such as feet, elbows and knees. Oilier and normal skins benefit from lotions, while oils and creams suit drier skins.

Exfoliating scrubs

Help combat the rough patches and blackheads that can appear on your skin by using a scrub. Use once or twice a week in the bath or shower, rinsing away the excess with clear warm water.

Pumice stone

These stones, made from very porous volcanic rock, work best if you lather up with soap before rubbing at hardened areas of skin in a circular motion. Don't rub too fiercely or else you'll make the skin sore. A little and often is best.

Loofahs and back brushes

Back brushes or long loofahs are useful as exfoliators, and their length makes them great for scrubbing difficult-to-reach areas like the back. Loofahs are actually the pod of an Egyptian plant and need a bit of care if they're to last. Rinse and drain them thoroughly after use to stop them going black and mouldy. Avoid rinsing them in vinegar and lemon juice as this can be too harsh for these once-living things. Back brushes are easier to care for; you simply rinse them in cool water after use and leave them to dry.

BATH TIME TREATS

Soaking in a warm bath has to be one of the most popular ways to relax. You can literally feel your cares disappear as you sink into the soothing water. However, you can also use bath time for a variety of other benefits and beauty boosters.

Learning to relax

Turn bathtime into an aromatherapy treat by adding relaxing essential oils such as chamomile and lavender to the water. Just add a few drops once you've run the bath, then lie back, inhale the vapours and relax. Salts and bubble baths that contain sea minerals and kelp also have a relaxing effect and purify your skin, too. Bathe by candlelight and listen to soothing music to make it even more of a treat. Put on eye pads and relax for 10 minutes.

BE A NATURAL BEAUTY

You don't have to splash out on expensive bath additives – try making your own:

■ Soothe irritated skin by adding a cup of cider vinegar to the running water.

■ A cup of powdered milk will soothe rough skin.

■ Add a cupful of oatmeal or bran to cleanse, whiten and soothe your skin.

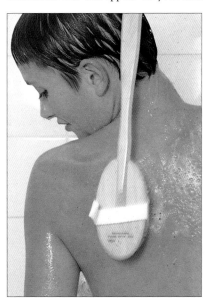

Above: Get back to basics with a brush to reach difficult areas.

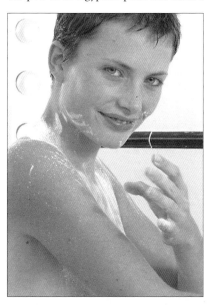

Above: Powder power for fresh, dry skin.

Sleek skin

Smooth your body with body oil before getting into the bath. After soaking for 10 minutes, rub your skin with a soft washcloth – you'll be amazed at how much dead skin you remove.

Boosting benefits

If you pat yourself dry after a bath, it'll help you to unwind, whereas briskly rubbing your skin with a towel will help to invigorate you.

SHOWER TIME TREATS

Showers are a wonderful opportunity to cleanse your body quickly, cheaply and to wake yourself up. Here are some of the other benefits.

Circulation booster

Switch on the cold water before finishing your shower to help boost your circulation. Strangely, it will also make you feel warmer once you get out of the shower. It also works well if you concentrate the blasts of cold water on cellulite-prone areas, as this stimulates the sluggish circulation in these spots.

Right: Splish! Splash! Relax and have fun in the bath.

Below: Turn a daily shower into a real power shower.

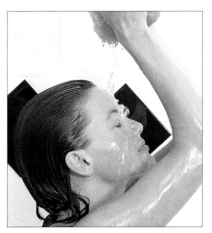

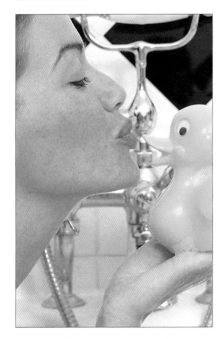

Above: Bath time is more fun if you share it.

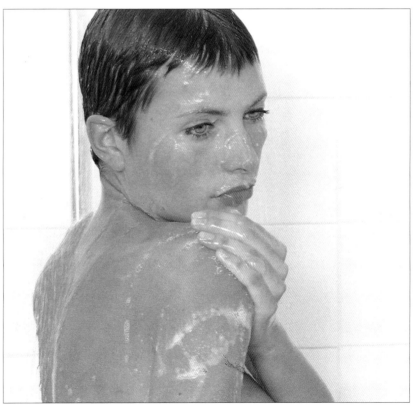

Your Bodycare Routine

When your mind is fixed on fast improvement, it is important to think about taking care of your whole body. For example, rough, mottled skin detracts from an otherwise great figure, but if it's smooth it will improve a not-so-perfect figure – and make a good one look even better.

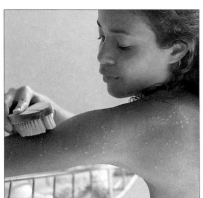

1 Body brushes can be used in the water. Do not use so vigorously that you damage the skin.

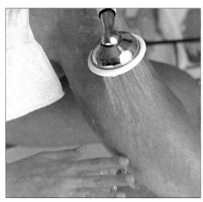

3 After exfoliating, spritz the skin with intermittent bursts of warm and then cool water to boost circulation and skin tone.

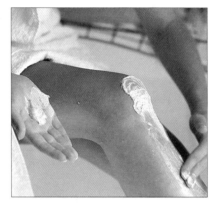

2 Remember to exfoliate the skin on your legs for all-over smoothness.

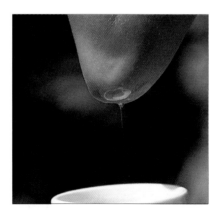

4 After spritzing, moisturize your skin. Oil is particularly nourishing for dry skin.

Your Basic Routine

Include the following steps in your bathroom routine and your skin will probably improve dramatically within a few weeks.

Body brush

Brushing your skin – from feet to hips and hands to shoulders – with a natural bristle brush exfoliates and tones. Go gently at first as you might find that your skin feels a bit tender to begin with. However, if you continue using a body brush each day you should be able to build up pressure and your skin will feel less sensitive over time. After body brushing these areas, take a little time to soak in a warm, oily bath to wind down and relax.

Exfoliation

Body exfoliators have larger grains than facial ones because body skin is tougher. It is easiest to buff in a shower or sauna. Try it – once a week or whenever you have time – on areas that are prone to dry skin, such as your elbows, shins, heels, knees, and your hands.

Moisturizing

Pay special attention to thirsty shins, elbows, upper arms, hips and knees; moisturize when your body is slightly damp and warm as creams will sink into the skin much more quickly.

Right: Dry areas such as shins and knees need lots of care, especially during the winter when cold weather removes natural moisture from the skin.

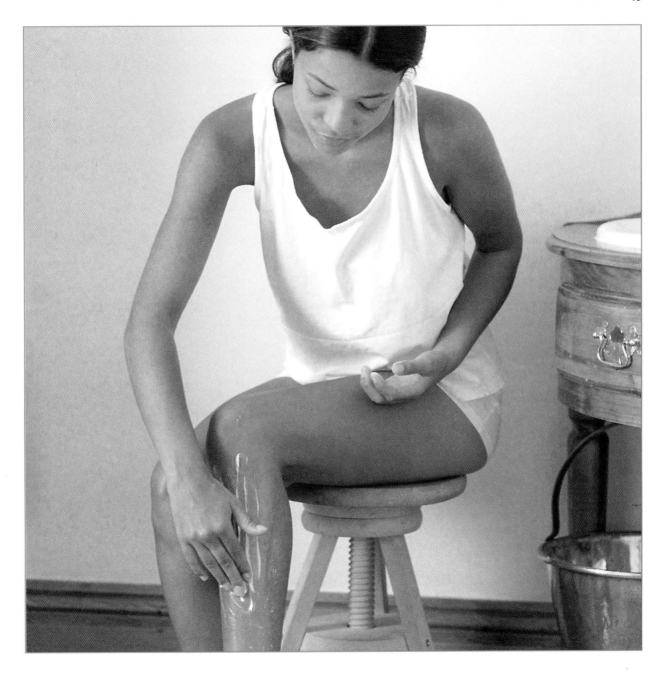

Caring for your Hands and Feet

Most of us do not give our hands and feet the attention they deserve. Our hands are constantly exposed to the elements, to harsh detergents, soaps and hot washing-up water. When our feet hit the ground they absorb nearly five times our body weight — it is important to remember to look after them.

CARING FOR YOUR HANDS

Hands are always visible, so the ideal is to have smooth skin and nicely manicured nails. But our hands are always exposed to the elements. This exposure causes the skin on the backs of our hands to age quickly; liver spots – pigmentation marks that look like oversized freckles – can appear, but these can be lightened with fading creams. To keep the skin on your hands supple, have a bottle of hand lotion by the kitchen sink and, if you dislike wearing rubber gloves, smother your hands with it before putting them into washing-up water or doing any other kind of housework.

Super-supple skin boosters

Manicurists treat hands that are dry to the point of cracking and callousing with skin-softening warm paraffin wax – the skin is coated with it and then peeled off when set. You can renourish really dry hands at home by soaking them in warm olive oil. Fill a teacup with the warmed oil, dip in your fingers and let them soak for a few minutes. When you remove them, rub the oil into your hands.

> **Lemon clean**
> Bleach stained hands naturally using fresh lemon juice; wash them afterwards with mild, unscented soap, and use a pumice stone to remove rough skin; then rub in lots of rich hand cream.

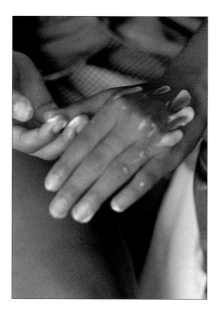

Above: Gently massage hand cream into your hands, remembering to rub it into the skin around the nails. Remove excess with a tissue.

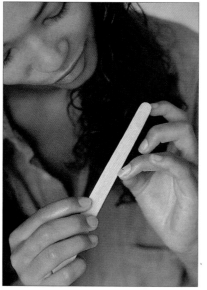

Above: Fingernails should be filed regularly. To minimize breakage, file them straight across with a soft emery board.

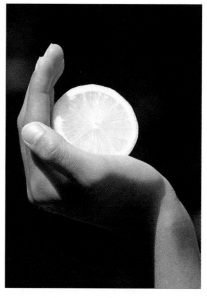

Above: The juice of a lemon is a good natural bleach for both hands and nails.

CARING FOR YOUR FEET

If you take care of your feet – keeping toenails trimmed, removing rough skin, and massaging feet and ankles regularly – you should not have any problems. This simple footcare routine does not take long – enjoy it a couple of times a week.

■ Remove any hard skin with a pumice stone or sloughing cream. If you use a foot file, rub your skin very gently before rinsing off the flaky residue.

■ Dry your feet well, especially between your toes; trim your toenails by cutting straight across the tip (but not down the sides), and file sharp corners with an emery board.

■ Soak your feet for a minimum of five minutes in a bowl or tub of hot water to which you have added some mineral salts or plain sea salt. Bubble foot spas are a good treat for feet; add a couple of drops of lavender essential oil to soothe aches and ease swelling.

■ Massage your feet by cupping your hands on either side of your foot and, using your thumbs, firmly pressing the upper part of your foot while pushing your thumbs down and outwards to the sides of your foot. Grasp each ankle and gently massage the ankle bone in circular movements to ease any stiffness. Work each foot in turn.

■ If your feet are feeling tired or swollen, try resting your feet above your head for 10 minutes. Do this by lying at right angles to a wall, or on the floor with your feet resting on the edge of a chair. Any swelling will disappear as trapped fluids travel back up your legs towards your heart.

Corn cures

Never try to tackle a corn yourself with a foot file, but go to a chiropodist. Soaking your feet in warm, soapy water will help to soften corns, and padded rings – which you can buy from a pharmacist – will ease the pressure.

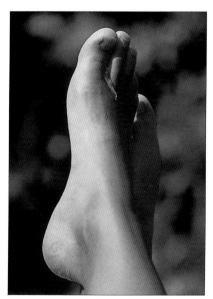

Above: After a long winter it may come as a shock to reveal your feet; it's important to keep the skin on your feet nourished and smooth.

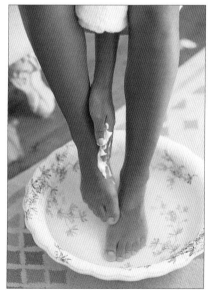

Above: To soften and remove dry skin, first soak your feet in warm water and cleanse thoroughly. Then use a foot file or pumice stone to remove the dry skin.

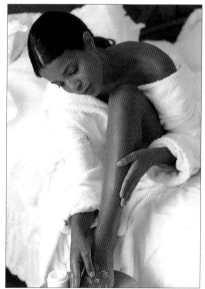

Above: After you have gently filed your feet with a foot file, smooth on foot cream to nourish and further soften the skin on your feet.

Scrub your Way to Smoother Skin

Improve your skin tone from head to toe with the regular use of a body scrub. This quick treatment is easy to do and boasts great results. The chances are, even if your skin isn't prone to spottiness or flaky patches, it will suffer from dullness and poor condition from time to time. This is where body scrubs and exfoliators come into their own. They work by shifting dead cells from the surface of your skin, revealing the younger, fresher ones underneath. This process also stimulates the circulation of blood in the skin tissues, giving it a rosy glow.

METHODS TO TRY

There are lots of different ways you can exfoliate your body – so there's one to suit every budget and preference.

▧ An exfoliating scrub is a cream- or gel-based product containing tiny abrasive particles. Use the type with rounded particles, which won't scratch and irritate delicate skin. Simply massage the scrub into damp skin, then rinse away thoroughly with lots of warm water.

▧ A bath mitt, loofah or sisal mitt are a cinch to use and cost effective, too. They can be quite harsh on the skin if you press too hard, so go easy at first. Simply sweep over your body when you're in the shower or bath. Rinse them well after use, and allow them to dry naturally.

▧ Your ordinary washcloth or bath sponge can also double up as an exfoliator. Lather up with plenty of soap or shower gel, and massage over damp skin before rinsing away with clear water.

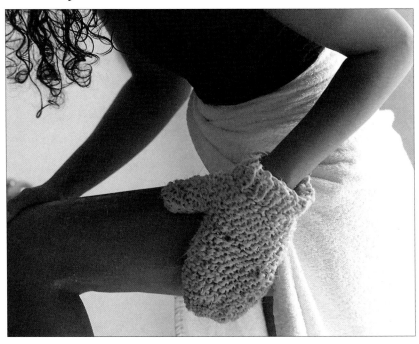

Above: Keep a sisal mitt to hand for super soft skin.

▧ Copy what health spas do, and keep a large tub of natural sea salt by the shower. Scoop up a handful when you get in, and massage over your skin. Rinse away thoroughly afterwards.

▧ Make your own body scrub by mixing sea salt with body oil or olive oil. Allow the mixture to soak into your skin for a few minutes to allow the edges of the salt to dissolve before massaging in. Rinse throughly with plenty of water.

▧ Body brushes are also useful. The best way to use them is on dry skin before you get in the bath or shower, as this is particularly good for loosening dead skin cells. You can also use them in the water, lathering them up with soap or gel. Try building up pressure gradually over several weeks. Just take care that you don't get too enthusiastic with the brushing and scrub your skin so vigorously that it becomes tender and sore.

Tip
For super-soft skin fast, you should massage your body with oil first before getting into the bath or shower. Then follow the exfoliating method you prefer.

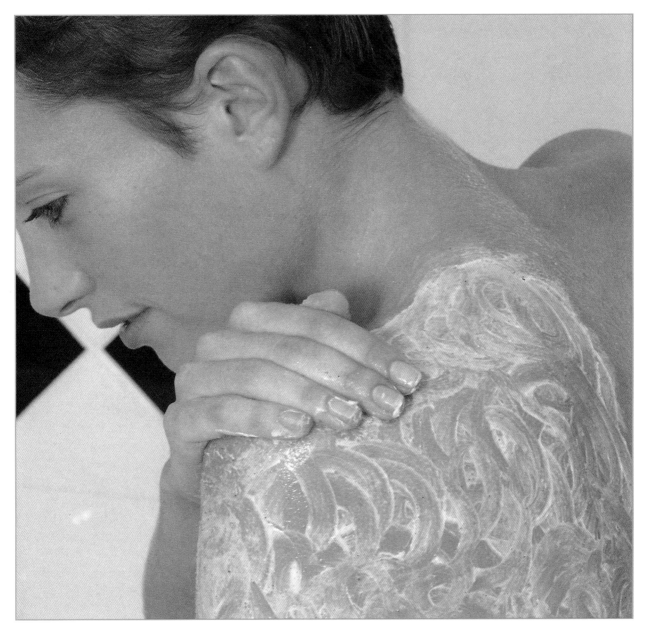

Above: Regular exfoliating works!

Simple Steps to Softer Skin

Slick on a body moisturizer to create a wonderfully silky body. Add a moisturizing body treat every day to your beauty regime, and you will soon reap the benefits.

MOISTURIZING MATTERS

Just as you choose a moisturizer for your face with care, you should opt for the best formulation suited to the skin type on your body.

■ Gels are the lightest formulation and are perfect for very hot days or oilier skin types. They contain a lot of nourishing ingredients even though they're very easy to wear.

■ Lotions and oils are good for most skin types. They are also easy to apply, as they're not too sticky.

■ Creams give better results for those with dry skins, especially very dry areas.

BODY MOISTURIZING

Here are a few tips to help you make the most of moisturizing your body.

■ Apply using firm strokes to boost your circulation as you massage in the product.

■ Apply the moisturizer straight onto clean, damp skin – after a bath or shower is the ideal time. This helps to seal moisture into the upper layers of your skin.

■ Soften cracked feet by rubbing them with rich body lotion, pulling on a pair of cotton socks and heading for bed. They'll be beautifully soft by the next morning!

■ Concentrate on rubbing moisturizer into particularly dry areas, such as heels, knees and elbows. The calves of the legs are also very prone to dryness because there aren't many oil glands there.

■ If you don't have time to apply moisturizer after your bath, simply add a few drops of body oil to the water. When you step out of the bath, your skin will be coated with a fine film of nourishing oil. Remember to rinse the bath well afterwards to prevent you from slipping the next time you take a dip.

■ Your breasts don't have any supportive muscle from the nipple to the collarbone and the skin is very fine here. Using firming creams and body lotions regularly won't work miracles, but they can help maintain the elasticity and suppleness in this delicate area.

Smelling scentsational

Opt for a scented body lotion as a wonderful treat. Applied as a lotion, the scent can be longer lasting than the actual fragrances themselves. Alternatively, use them as part of "fragrance layering". This simply means taking advantage of the various scent formulations that are now available. Start with a scented bath oil and soap, move onto the matching body lotion and powder, and leave the house wearing the fragrance itself sprayed onto pulse points.

However, be careful you don't clash fragrances. Opt for unscented products if you're also wearing a perfume, unless you're going to be wearing a matching scented body lotion. You don't want a whole range of cheaper products competing or clashing with your more expensive perfume.

Above: Opt for the light touch with a moisturizing gel.

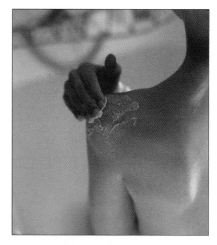

Above: Shoulders and upper arms benefit from exfoliation before moisturizing.

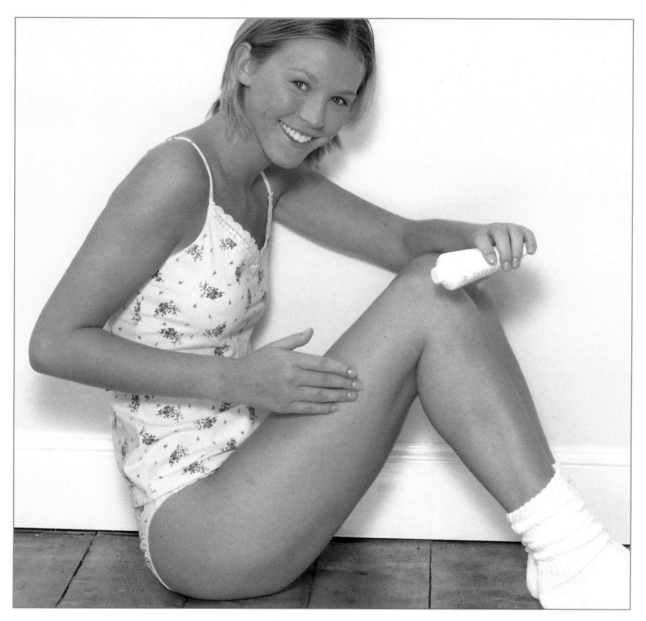

Above: Take the time before dressing to moisturize your skin. Why not apply body lotion and then let your skin absorb it whilst you clean your teeth or dry your hair?

Indulge yourself with Aromatherapy

Aromatherapy is one of the most popular therapies around today. It's wonderful to use, the products are easily available, and they can provide you with immediate results. Aromatherapy uses essential oils, which are distilled essences of herbs, plants, flowers and trees. Most of these oils smell wonderful and are a pleasure to use. It's this smell that usually attracts people to them for treating a variety of physical and mental conditions, from skin infections to stress. There are three main ways to use essential oils.

In the bath

Add 5-10 drops of your chosen oil to your bath, then sink in and relax. Inhaling the wonderful aromas will soothe your mind, and the oils will also have a beneficial effect on your skin and body. Only pour oil into the bath once it's started to run, or the oil will evaporate with the heat of the water and you'll lose the therapeutic properties of the essential oil before you even get in.

For massage

Mix 3-4 drops of essential oil into 10 ml (2 teaspoons) of neutral carrier oil, such as sweet almond oil, and use to massage your body – or ask someone else to massage you. Alternatively, choose one of the many pre-blended oils currently available on the market. Most aromatherapists believe that you're naturally drawn to the oils that will do you most good at that time.

To perfume your room

Fragrance your room and indulge in the beneficial scent. Clay burners are readily available to diffuse oils into the air. Add the oil to some water in the bowl at the top, then light the night candle underneath. Using the water as a carrier for the essential oil will prevent the oil from burning and help to create sweet-smelling steam to permeate your room. Alternatively, place six drops of your chosen oil in a small bowl of water and put it in a warm place, such as on top of a radiator in winter. There are also ring diffusers you can put under light bulbs to very gently heat the oil, or you can add a few drops of oil to the water in a plant sprayer, and use it to spritz the room whenever you like.

Above: Flower power – treat yourself with fragrant oils from flowers, plants and herbs.

WONDERFUL OILS TO TRY

There are several hundred essential oils to choose from, so it can be confusing knowing which ones to try. These are some useful ones to start with:

Essential oil	Benefits	Use for
Chamomile	calming	headaches and anxiety
Mandarin	calming, refreshing	digestive problems
Eucalyptus	decongestant	colds
Lavender	calming and balancing	stress, colds, headaches, PMT
Peppermint	refreshing	indigestion and sickness
Rose	soothing	depression
Rosemary	antiseptic and stimulating	aches and pains
Sandalwood	relaxing	stress, dry skin care
Tea tree	anti-bacterial	pimples and cold sores
Ylang ylang	love potion	boosting sex drive

AROMATHERAPY TIPS

1 If you don't want to buy individual essential oils buy them ready-blended, or treat yourself to bath and body products that contain them.

2 Some oils are thought to carry some risk during pregnancy. For this reason, consult a qualified aromatherapist for advice if you are expecting a child and want to use essential oils.

3 Don't try to treat medical conditions with them – always consult your doctor.

4 Essential oils can be expensive, but remember that a little goes a long way.

5 Don't apply essential oils to the skin undiluted as they are far too concentrated in this form, and can result in inflammation. The only exception is lavender, which can be used directly on the skin for insect bites and stings. Otherwise essential oils should be mixed with a carrier oil.

6 Don't take essential oils internally. Essential oils are approximately 50-100 times more powerful than the plant they were extracted from.

7 Don't apply oils to areas of broken, inflamed or recently scarred skin.

8 Whichever method of aromatherapy you use, shut the door to the room to prevent the aroma from escaping.

9 For immediate results from aromatherapy, try inhaling the steam. Add about four drops of your chosen oil to a bowl of hot water, lean over it and cover your head with a towel. Inhale deeply for about five minutes.

10 Place a few drops of your favourite oil on a tissue, so you can inhale it whenever you like. Eucalyptus is great if your sinuses are blocked or you have a cold. A few drops of chamomile or lavender on your pillow will help you sleep.

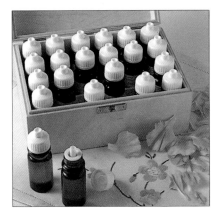

Above: Special essential oils - for a sensual experience.

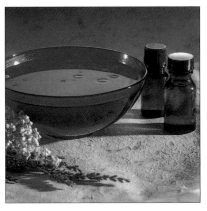

Above: Put a few drops of essential oils into hot water and inhale the steam.

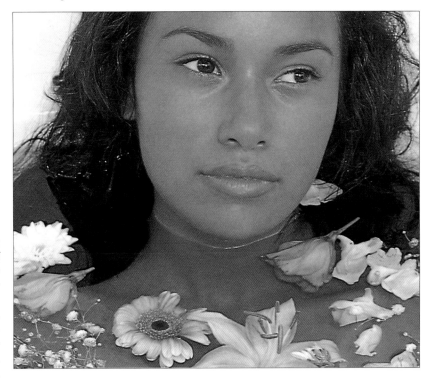

Above: Try a soothing aromatherapy bath, and let your cares float away.

Beat the Cellulite Problem

It's not just plumper, older women who suffer from "orange-peel skin" on their thighs, hips, bottom and even tummy – many slim, young women suffer, too. Despite what you may have heard, there is no miracle cure for cellulite, but there are some effective and practical things you can do to see great results.

FACTS ON CELLULITE

Experts differ about what exactly causes cellulite. It seems likely that it's an accumulation of fat, fluid and toxins trapped into the hardened network of elastin and collagen fibres in the deeper levels of the skin. This causes the dimpled effect and feel of cellulite areas. These areas also tend to feel cold to the touch because the flow of blood is constricted and the lymph system, which is responsible for eliminating toxins, can't work properly. This can worsen the problem and make the cellulite feel puffy and spongy.

HAVE I GOT CELLULITE?

Try squeezing the skin or your upper thigh between your thumb and index finger. If the flesh feels lumpy and looks bumpy, you have cellulite. Further clues may be that these areas look whiter, and feel colder than elsewhere on your legs.

Common causes

Cellulite can be caused and/or aggravated by the following:

■ Hereditary factors – if your mother has cellulite, it's a fair bet you will have, too.

■ Hormones, such as the contraceptive pill, may be contributory.

■ A poor diet is full of toxins and puts the body under great strain to get rid of vast quantities of waste. Also, an unhealthy low-fibre, high-fat diet means that the body's digestive system can't work effectively to expel toxins from the body.

■ Stress and lack of exercise make your body sluggish and can slow down blood circulation and the lymphatic system.

TAKING THE SENSIBLE APPROACH

There are dozens of products around designed to deal with cellulite, but to really tackle the problem you should follow a three-pronged approach, combining:

■ Circulation-boosting tactics
■ Diet
■ Exercise

BOOST YOUR CIRCULATION

Here are several ways to boost your circulation and your lymphatic system. Whichever one you choose, aim to follow it for at least five minutes a day.

■ Use a massage glove or rough sisal mitt to stimulate your skin.

Make your own cellulite cream

Some women swear by aromatherapy to treat their cellulite. There are many ready-blended oils on the market, but you can make your own. Just add two drops each of rosemary and fennel essential oils to three teaspoons of carrier oil, such as almond oil. Massage this mixture daily thoroughly into the affected areas.

■ Use a soft body brush on damp or dry skin, brushing in long, sweeping movements over the afflicted area, and working in the direction of the heart.

■ Use a cellulite cream. These usually contain natural ingredients such as horse chestnut and ivy to pep up your circulation. However, you can make them doubly effective by massaging them in with your fingers. Some cellulite creams come with their own plastic or rubber hand-held mitts to help boost the circulation.

■ Some women find that aromatherapy helps to reduce their cellulite. There are many ready-blended oils on the market.

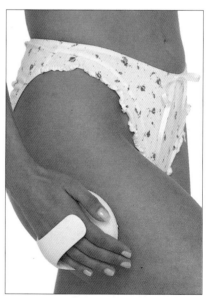

Above: Pep up your circulation and lymphatic system daily to help beat that cellulite.

STEP UP YOUR EXERCISE

Exercise will boost your sluggish circulation and lymphatic system. It will also encourage your body to get rid of the toxins causing your cellulite. Do a regular aerobic workout, exercising for 20-40 minutes, between three and five times a week, and choose from these: brisk walking, jogging, swimming, cycling, tennis, badminton, aerobic classes or running. (It is always wise to consult your doctor before embarking on a new form of exercise.)

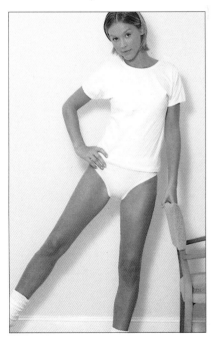

Hip toner

Stand sideways with your hand resting on a chair. Your knees should be slightly bent and your shoulders relaxed. Slowly raise your right leg, keeping your body and raised foot facing forward. Carefully and slowly lower your leg, and then repeat this movement at least 10 times. Then turn round and repeat the exercise with the other leg.

Tone it up!

You can also try these exercises to firm up your legs and give them a better shape. Carried out daily, they will help you win the cellulite battle.

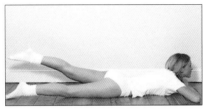

Bottom toner

Lie on your front with your hands on top of one another, resting your chin on them if you wish. Raise one leg about 13 cm (5 in) off the floor, and hold for a count of 10. Bring your leg back to the floor, and repeat 15-20 times with each leg.

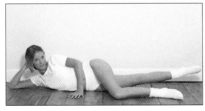

Inner thigh toner

Lie on your side on the floor. With your top leg resting on the floor in front, raise the lower leg off the floor as far as you can without straining, then gently lower it again. Repeat 10 times, then turn over and work the other leg.

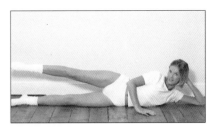

Outer thigh toner

Lie on your side, supporting your head with your hand. Bend your lower leg behind you and tilt your hips slightly forward. Place your other hand on the floor in front of you for balance. Slowly lift your upper leg, then bring it down to touch the lower one, and repeat this action at least six times. Repeat on the other side.

FOLLOW A DETOX DIET

To detoxify your body you need to follow a healthy low-fat, high-fibre diet – one that contains plenty of fresh fruit and vegetables. The great news is, if you have any excess weight to lose it will naturally fall away by following these rules.

■ Eat at least five servings of fresh fruit and vegetables every day.

■ Cut down on the amount of fat you eat. For instance, grill rather than fry foods, and cut off visible fat from meat.

■ Water cleanses your system and flushes toxins from body cells, so drink at least two litres (quarts) of pure water every day.

■ Change from caffeine-laden tea and coffee to herbal teas and decaffeinated coffee. Sip pure fruit juices rather than fizzy drinks.

Brownie Points in the Sun

There's nothing that lifts your spirits like spending time in the sunshine. However, you need to take special care of your skin against the potential dangers of suntanning.

KNOW YOUR SPFS

The initials SPF stand for Sun Protection Factor. The higher the number of the SPF, the more protection the product will give you from the burning ultraviolet B (UVB) rays. To decide which SPF suits you, you need to know how vulnerable your skin is to the sun's UVB rays. Dermatologists divide skins into the following six types.

Skin type 1

Always burns, never tans. Fair-skinned, usually with freckles. Red or blonde hair. Typical Anglo-Saxon or Irish skin type.
UK/North Europe: Total sunblock.
USA/Tropics/Africa: Total sunblock.
Mediterranean: Total sunblock.

Skin type 2

Burns easily and tans with difficulty. Fair hair and pale skin. Typical North European skin type.
UK/North Europe: Start with SPF 20 and use sunblock on delicate areas. Progress gradually to SPF 15.
USA/Tropics/Africa: Start with sunblock and progress gradually to SPF 20.
Mediterranean: Start with SPF 20 and use sunblock on delicate areas. Progress gradually to SPF 15.

Skin type 3

Sometimes burns but tans well. Light brown hair and medium skin-tone. A typical North European skin type.
UK/North Europe: Start with SPF 10 and progress to SPF 8.
USA/Tropics/Africa: Start with SPF 20, moving to SPF 15, then SPF 10.
Mediterranean: Start with SPF 15, moving to SPF 10.

Skin type 4

Occasionally burns but tans easily. Usually with brown hair and eyes, and olive skin. The typical Mediterranean skin type.
UK/North Europe: Start with SPF 8, moving to SPF 6.
USA/Tropics/Africa: Start with SPF 15, moving to SPF 8.
Mediterranean: Start with SPF 10, moving to SPF 6.

Skin type 5

Hardly ever burns and tans easily. Dark eyes, dark hair and olive skin. A typical Middle Eastern or Asian skin type.
UK/North Europe: Use SPF 6.
USA/Tropics/Africa: Start with SPF 8 and move to SPF 6.
Mediterranean: Start SPF 8, and move to SPF 6.

Skin type 6

Almost never burns. Dark hair, eyes, and skin. A typical African or Afro-Caribbean skin type.
UK/North Europe: No sunscreen is needed.
USA/Tropics/Africa: Start with SPF 8 and move to SPF 6.
Mediterranean: Use SPF 6 throughout.

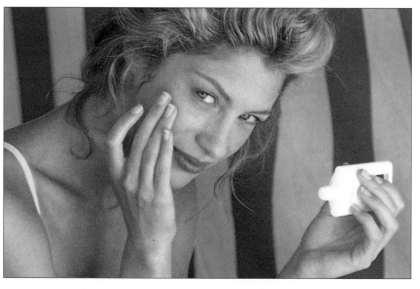

Above: Protect and survive. Guard against ageing and the burning rays of the sun with an effective sun cream.

YOUR SAFE TAN PLAN

■ Apply suntan lotion (block) before you go into the sun and before you dress, to ensure that you don't miss any areas.

■ Gradually build up the time you spend in the sun. Never be tempted to burn – it's a sign of skin damage.

■ Stay out of the sun between 12 noon and 3 o'clock when the sun is at its hottest. Move into the shade or cover up with a T-shirt and broad-brimmed hat.

■ If you're playing a lot of sports or swimming, choose a special sports formula or waterproof formulation.

■ Lips need a good lip screen to protect them from burning and chapping.

■ Like skincare ranges, there are hypoallergenic suncare products around, so ask at your pharmacist.

JOIN THE BROWNIES – WITH A FAKE TAN

The safest tan of all is one that comes out of a bottle. There are three main ways to fake a tan.

Bronzing powders

Use powders on your face in the same way as a blusher. Make sure that the one you use is not too pearlized, or you'll really shimmer in the sunshine.

Wash-off tanners

This is the simplest way to create an instant tan on your face and body. You simply smooth on the cream and then wash it away at the end of the day.

Self tanners

Formulations contain an active ingredient called dihydroxyacetone (DHA), which is absorbed by the surface skin cells and turns brown in the presence of oxygen – which creates the "tan". This process usually takes three to four hours, and the effects last until these skin cells are naturally shed – which can be from a few days up to a week. Self tanners make an acceptable alternative to the real thing.

SELF-TANNING TIPS

■ Use a body scrub first to rub away the dead flaky skin that can soak up colour and create a patchy finish.

■ Massage in plenty of body lotion over the area to be treated. This will combat any remaining dry areas and give a smooth surface on which to apply the tanning lotion.

■ If there's a shade choice, go with the lighter one, because you can always apply a second layer later on.

■ Work the product firmly into the skin until it feels completely dry. Any excess left on the surface is likely to go patchy.

■ If you've applied self tanner to your body, wipe areas that don't normally tan with damp cotton wool pads (cotton balls) – armpits, nipples, soles of feet and fingers. On the face, work the cotton wool around eyebrows, hairline and jawline.

■ While there are self-tanning products that offer some protection from the sun until you wash your skin, it's best to use them in conjunction with the best sunscreen for your skin type.

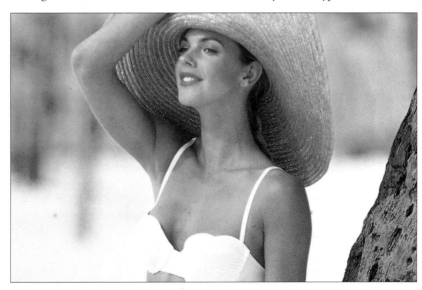

Above: Go for the glow with a light tan.

Your Top Skincare Questions

1 Night watch

Q "My dry skin needs night cream, but I seem to lose most of it onto my pillow. Any solutions?"

A Put a little night cream into the palm of your hand, then gently rub your hands together. The heat created will help liquefy the cream and make it more easily absorbed. Gently massage it into your skin, and you'll find it sinks in better. Another method is to place the cream in a teaspoon, and heat gently over a low gas flame on the cooker until just warm, before applying as usual. It sounds strange, but it really works.

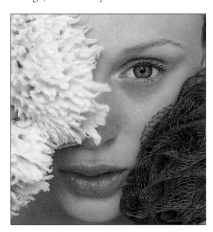

Above: The soft touch of a sponge or facecloth is a cheap – and effective – option to a facial scrub.

2 Polished perfection

Q "I spend a fortune on skincare products, but resent paying for an exfoliator. Are there any alternatives?"

A Yes, here's a good, cheap alternative to facial scrubs. After washing your skin, gently massage with a soft facecloth or natural sponge to ease away the dead surface skin cells that can give your complexion a muddy look. Make sure you avoid ones with scratchy surfaces as they'll be too harsh for your skin. If you have dry skin, massage a little cream cleanser onto damp skin, then rub over the top with your flannel (wash cloth). Rinse afterwards, then apply moisturizer in the normal way. It is essential to wash the facecloth after every couple of uses and to hang it up to dry in between to prevent the build-up of bacteria.

3 Lip tricks

Q "How can I stop my lips from getting so chapped and flaky in winter?"

A This three-step action plan will help.

■ Massage dry lips with a generous dollop of petroleum jelly. Allow it to work for a couple of minutes to soften your skin. Then, gently rub your lips with a warm, damp facecloth. As the petroleum jelly is removed, the flakes of skin will come with it.

■ Smooth your lips morning and night with a lip balm.

■ Switch to a moisturizing lipstick to prevent your lips from drying out during the daytime.

4 Red nose day

Q "It's so embarrassing! My nose looks really red in the winter. What's the best way to cover it?"

A Try smoothing a little green foundation or concealer over the red area before applying your normal foundation and powder. Although it sounds strange, the green works by cancelling out the redness – leaving your skin looking a normal shade again.

5 Winter sun

Q "Someone told me you should still wear a sunscreen in winter. Is this true?"

A Yes, if you want to guard against the signs of ageing. Exposure to sunlight is thought to be the main cause of wrinkling, and the ultraviolet rays that are responsible for this process are around every single day of the year. You don't, however, need to use a suntan lotion – just choose one of the many moisturizers that contain sunscreens.

6 Lighten up

Q "My skin feels as though it needs a richer cream in the winter months, but I find most of them too heavy. What can you suggest?"

A Choose the level of moisturizer that feels right for you. Just because moisturizer is heavier, it doesn't necessarily mean

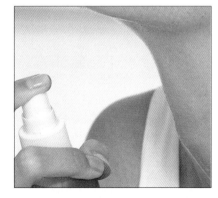

Above: Puttin' on the spritz – boost the moisture in your skin by spraying with water before moisturizing.

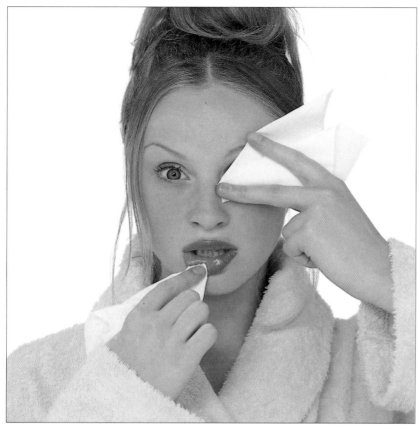

Left: Remove all traces of make-up before going to bed.

8 Sensitive issue

Q "Why does my skin feel more sensitive in winter than summer?"

A Eighty per cent of women claim to have sensitive skin – which tingles, itches and is prone to dryness. It can be aggravated by harsh winter weather, such as the winds and cold, because this breaks down the natural oily layer which protects your skin. Milder summer weather doesn't tend to be so hard on the skin. The best way to cope is to moisturize your skin regularly with a hypoallergenic cream that is specially formulated for sensitive skin.

9 Pregnant pause

Q "I'm pregnant and have developed patches of darker colour on my face, particularly under my eyes and around my mouth. What causes this?"

A This is called chloasma, or "the mask of pregnancy". It's triggered by a change in hormones at this time and is made more obvious by sunbathing. Cover up under the sun and wear a sunblock to prevent the patches from becoming denser. It usually fades within a few months of having your baby. Chloasma can also be triggered by the contraceptive pill, but disappears again once you stop taking them.

10 On the spot

Q "I suffer from oily skin, but find blemish creams too drying. What can you suggest?"

A Many women have skin that has dry patches as well as blemishes. The solution is to choose an antibacterial cream that

it's more effective. You can help seal in extra moisture to your skin by spritzing your complexion with water before applying it. Also, choose a nourishing foundation or tinted moisturizer to ensure that your skin stays smooth and soft all day long. You can help counteract the drying effects of central heating by placing a bowl of water near the radiators to replenish the moisture levels in the air.

7 Water factor

Q "I like the feeling of water on my face, but I find soap too drying. Should I switch to a cream cleanser instead?"

A If you have dry skin, it's generally better to use a creamy cleanser, which you apply with your fingertips and remove with cotton wool pads (cotton balls) or soft tissues. This will prevent too much moisture from being lost from the surface of your skin. However, normal and oily skins can still happily use water – but switch to a facial wash or wash-off cleanser instead. They're specially formulated to be non-drying, while still getting your face clean – and you can splash with water as much as you like!

will kill off the cause of your blemishes, while soothing the skin around them. This means you won't be left with dry patches of skin as well as blemishes.

11 Treatment sprays

Q " I find body lotions too hot and sticky to wear after bathing. Is there anything else I can try?"
A There's a lovely new trend for body treatment sprays, which combine the moisturizing and toning properties of a body care product with the fragrance of a traditional perfume. This means they'll make you smell beautifully fresh as well as lightly moisturize your skin. Many of the large perfume companies now offer a choice of these products.

12 The throat vote

Q "The skin on my neck looks grey and dull. Are there any special treatments I can use?"
A Necks can quickly shown the signs of ageing. This is mainly due to the fact that they have a lack of sebaceous glands. Using a creamy cleanser can help. Massage in, leave to dissolve dirt, and then remove with cotton wool pads (cotton balls). Dull grey skin will benefit from regular exfoliation – scrub briskly with a facecloth or soft shaving brush. Grey lines on the neck and throat can be bleached away by smoothing plain yogurt over clean skin. Leave on for about half an hour, then rinse away thoroughly with warm water. Boost softness by smoothing on moisturizer. Your ordinary cream moisturizer will do the job.

13 Beautiful back

Q "How can I get rid of the pimples on my back and bottom?"

A Because backs are covered up and hard to reach, they're prone to breakouts. Keep yours blemish free by exfoliating daily with a loofah or body brush to remove dry, flaking skin and superficial blemishes. For more stubborn pimples, try a clay mask to draw out deep-seated impurities. Smooth onto broken-out areas, leave until dry, then rinse away with lots of warm water.

14 Mole watch

Q "I understand you need to keep an eye on moles on your skin to guard against the risk of skin cancer. But what exactly should I be looking for?"
A Moles are clumps of clustered pigment cells that are nearly always darker than freckles. All changes in existing moles

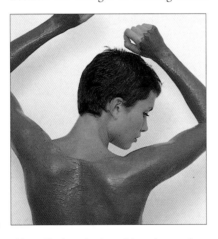

Above: Back to basics with a clay mask for the body.

should be checked by your doctor. Any that cause concern will be removed and sent off for analysis. You should also check moles yourself once a month. Try the following ABCD Code: check for A

(asymmetry); B (border irregularity); C (colour change); D (change in diameter).

15 Shadow sense

Q "I've got dark shadows under my eyes. What's the best way to deal with them?"
A Dark shadows can be the result of a variety of causes, including fatigue, anaemia, poor digestion and lack of fresh air. They can also be hereditary. If in doubt, consult your doctor for advice. Take steps to ensure that you're cutting out the causes – for instance, getting a good night's sleep and keeping to a low-fat, high-fibre diet.

For special occasions, you can bathe the area with pads soaked in ice-cold water for 15 minutes. This will help lessen the shadow effect temporarily. Or cover shadows by dotting on some concealer over the affected area.

16 Brown baby

Q "Is there anything I can do to hang on to my tan for longer?"
A Just when you want to show off a golden tan, it begins to peel away. This is because your skin is especially dry after sunbathing, so it sheds its old cells more quickly. You can prolong the colour for a little while longer by applying lots of body lotion in the morning and evening. Apply it while your skin is still damp to make it extra effective. Apply a little fake tan every few days to keep your colour topped up. Or better still - protect your skin by not tanning at all.

17 Sticky situation

Q "I exercise a lot and find body odour a problem. How can I prevent it?"
A Sweating is your body's natural cooling device. Sweat itself has no odour, but it

begins to smell when it comes into contact with bacteria on the skin's surface. Keeping underarms hair-free can help prevent sweat from being trapped.

Opt for an antiperspirant deodorant rather than just an ordinary deodorant alone. The antiperspirants help prevent sweating, while the deodorant helps prevent odour. As a result, a product with the combination of the two is highly effective. Also, try to wear natural fibres next to your skin because they help you to stay fresh for longer.

18 Massage magic

Q "I had a facial massage in a beauty salon. Is there a way I can give myself one at home?"

A Yes, just like every other part of your body, your face will look better after a bit of exercise, and a massage is the ideal way to give your complexion a workout. Pour a few drops of vegetable oil into the palms of your hands and smooth it onto your face and neck. Make sure your skin is damp, as this makes the oil go on more easily. Then follow these steps:

■ Use your fingers to stroke upwards from the base of your neck to your chin.
■ Continue with long strokes up one side of your face, then the other.
■ Now go around your nose and up towards your forehead.
■ When you get to your forehead, stroke it across from left to right using one hand. Finish off by gently drawing a circle around each eye using one finger.

19 Stretch marks

Q "Is there anything I can do to get rid of the stretch marks that have appeared on my tummy, breasts and thighs?"

A There's little you can do once you've got them, except wait until they start to fade. However, keeping your skin well moisturized can help guard against getting them in the first place. An application of fake tan can be a good disguise for stretch marks that might be on view.

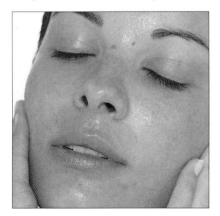

Above: Stroke away the strains and stresses of the day.

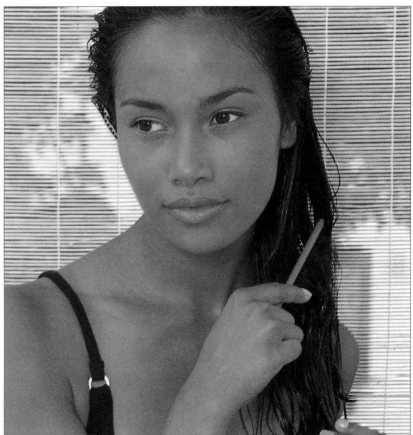

Above: Take time in the bathroom to pamper yourself from head to toe.

Beauty Buzzwords

If you're confused about the various claims and ingredients in your skincare products, check out what they mean here in your guide to the most commonly found skincare jargon.

Allergy-screened

Means that the individual ingredients in the product have gone through exacting tests to ensure that they're safe to use and that there's just the minimum risk of causing allergy.

Aloe vera

The juice from the leaves of this cactus-type plant is often used in skincare ingredients because of its soothing, protecting and moisturizing qualities.

Antioxidants

Work by mopping up and absorbing "free radicals" (highly reactive molecules that can damage your skin and cause premature ageing) from your skin. Good antioxidants are the ACE vitamins, i.e. vitamins A, C and E.

Benzoyl peroxide

An ingredient commonly used in over-the-counter spot and acne treatments. It gently peels surface skin and unclogs blocked follicles which can cause spots.

Cocoa butter

Comes from the seeds of the cacao tree in tropical climates. Cocoa butter is an excellent moisturizer, especially for dry skin on the body.

Right: A pH balanced facial wash will help prevent your skin feeling tight.

Collagen

An elastic type of substance in the underlying tissues of your skin that provide support and springiness. Collagen is a popular ingredient in skincare treatments, although it's doubtful if a molecule this size can actually penetrate the skin.

Dermatologically tested

Means the product has been patch tested on a panel of human volunteers to monitor it for any tendency to cause irritation. This means it's usually suitable for sensitive skins.

Elastin

Fibres in the underlying layer of your skin, rather like collagen, which help give it strength and elasticity.

Exfoliation

The whisking away of the top layers of dead surface cells from your skin, making it look brighter and feel smoother.

Fruit acids

These are also known as AHAs or alpha-hydroxy acids. They're commonly found in natural products, such as fruit, sour milk and wine. AHAs are included in many face creams because they work by breaking down the protein bonds that hold together the dead cells on the skin's surface, to reveal newer, fresher skin underneath.

Humectants

Are ingredients often found in moisturizers, as they work by attracting moisture to themselves, and so keep the surface layers of your skin well hydrated.

Hypoallergenic

These products are usually fragrance-free, contain the minimum of colouring agents and no known irritants or sensitizers. This is not a total guarantee that no one will have an allergic reaction to them. Some people are allergic to water.

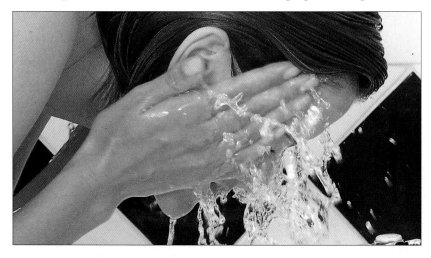

Jojoba oil

A gentle, non-irritant oil which makes an excellent moisturizer as it is easily absorbed into the skin and helps improve the condition of the hair and scalp.

Lanolin free

Means a product doesn't contain anolin. At one time it was thought that lanolin was a skin allergen, although evidence now seems to show that lanolin is even suitable for sensitive skins.

Liposomes

Tiny fluid-filled spheres of the same material that forms cell membranes. Their very small size is said to let them penetrate into the skin's living cells, where they act as delivery parcels that release their active ingredients.

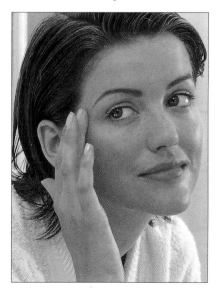

Above: Ensure your moisturizer has an effective sunscreen – check the SPF rating to be sure.

Milia

Another word for whiteheads – small pimples on the skin. Oil produced from the sebaceous glands gathers to form a white plug that is trapped under the skin. You can try to remove these by gently squeezing with tissue-covered fingers or treat them with an antibacterial cream.

Non-comedogenic

Means the product has been screened to eliminate ingredients which can clog the follicles and encourage blackheads and spots (a comedo is a blackhead). It's particularly useful for oily skins.

Oil of Evening Primrose

It is very useful for helping your skin retain its moisture. It's a wonderful moisturizer, particularly for dry or very dry skins, as it hydrates, protects and soothes. Many sufferers of eczema find it useful.

pH balanced

Refers to the pH scale, which measures the acidity or alkalinity of a solution. Seven means that it is neutral. Any number below that is acidic, and numbers above are alkaline. Healthy skin has a slightly acidic reading, so pH balanced skincare products are slightly acidic to maintain this natural optimum level.

SPF

Stands for Sun Protection Factor. It tells you how long the sun cream or moisturizer will protect you from the sun's ultraviolet B (UVB) rays. The higher the number, the more protection it gives you.

T-zone

The T-zone is the area across the forehead and down the centre of the face where the oil glands and sweat glands of the face are most concentrated.

Ultraviolet (UV) rays

UVB rays will burn and damage your skin if you sunbathe too long. UVA rays are strong all year round and cause ageing and wrinkling of the skin. Guard against this with a broad-spectrum sun cream, which contains both UVA and UVB filters to protect you year round.

Vitamin E

Often used in moisturizers because it can help combat dryness and the signs of ageing. It's also useful for helping to heal scars and burns.

Water soluble

Cleansers are described as water soluble when they contain oils to dissolve grime and make-up from the skin. They have the added bonus that they can be easily rinsed away from the skin with plenty of fresh, clean water.

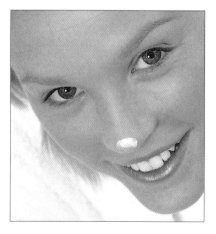

Above: Try the healing benefits of vitamin E on your skin.

Index

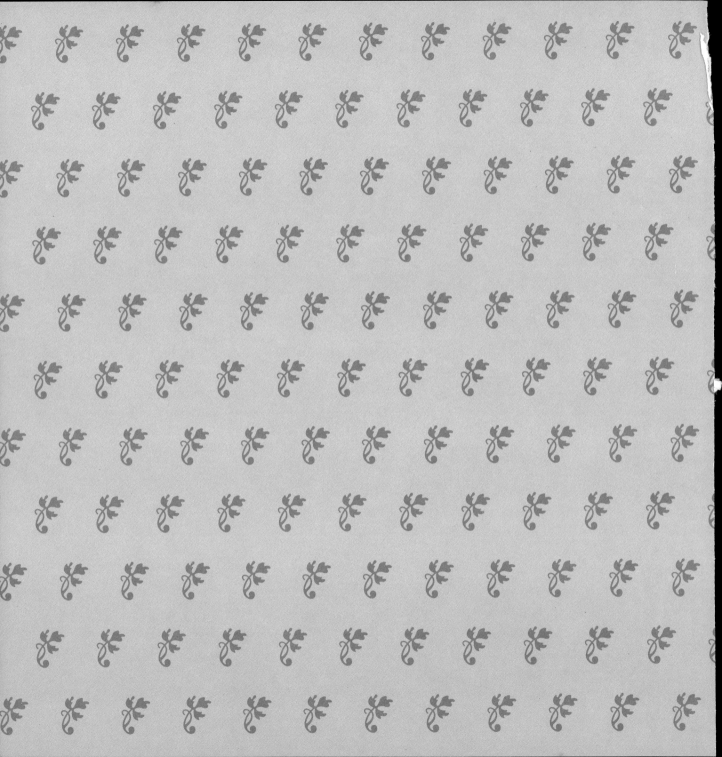